Every sick person
is
a God/Goddess who doesn't know it

I dedicate this book to all the sovereigns I have known, my former patients, for your confidence in me over the past twenty-five years. You taught me about life. It is with much gratitude that I submit this work to you.

As well, to all of my former collaborators, the staff of my clinics, for your loyalty and support. You enabled me to look beyond and explore new horizons. It is with much affection that I share my discoveries with you.

Thank you all from the bottom of my heart!

If your local bookstore is out, please contact
our sales office to order:

HERE'S THE KEY INC.

In the USA	In Canada
P.O. Box 223	P.O. Box 113
Morgan, VT	Coaticook, QC
05853	J1A 2S9
Tel: 1-802-895-4914	Tel: 1-819-835-9520
Fax: 1-802-895-4669	Fax: 1-819-835-5433

THE
MEDICAL
MAFIA

*How to get out of it alive and take back
our health & wealth*

by

Guylaine Lanctôt, M.D.

Table of contents

The trilogy of lies, part three:

The realization: *self-health*

Prologue

A HEART-TO-HEART TÊTE-À-TÊTE

This book is the fruit of medical studies, apprenticeship, learning by experience, and reflection over 25 years of practicing and being involved in the world of medicine.

To some, this work will seem obvious. To others, it will appear to be nonsense, an aberration. It will please one. And shock the other.

In part, it is with one's brain that one will **understand** this book. And, in part, it is with one's heart that one will **perceive** it. Certain areas are explored using logic, others thanks to intuition. My medical studies have taught me the importance of being rigorous, precise, accurate and statistically correct. Life has taught me, however, that it doesn't always work out as spelled out in the treatise or as written in stone. I am not going to express myself in an academic or didactic fashion. But rather I will **relate** to you what I have seen, read, understood, actually experienced, and concluded. I am going to avoid statistics which, after all, can prove whatever they set out to prove. I will restrict myself to presenting approximate ballpark figures with all the margin of error that they entail. Do not look for proof, footnotes, or exact figures. You will not find them. I am not a statistician, nor an archivist or journalist. Nor am I a professional researcher or economist. But common sense and love, that I know. My aim is not to convince you, but to **inform** you. Having said that:

- Either your inner voice will tell you that it is true and, therefore, you will not need any proof.
- Or, your inner voice will tell you that it is not true, and no amount of proof is going to convince you otherwise.
- Or your inner voice will cause you to question and want to know more, and I will cite books already full of references.

When I recommend these books for you to read, I am not necessarily endorsing the contents or the message. There are some that I have read from cover to cover. Others that I just flipped through. And others that I have not read at all. That is not important in the least. For it is you who will draw your own conclusions. I am happy only to inform you of their existence. The only truth that is of any consequence to you, is your own. If you know of other books which might help readers to better understand, would you be so kind as to let me know their titles.

It is the same with quotes. I include those that have caused me to reflect, hoping that they will do the same for you.

Despite its title, this book is not a denunciation of the medical world. Many others have already done that. I am not looking for a guilty party or a scapegoat. For who are we to judge others? Besides, I am not in a position to do that, given the fact that it is by having been a participant and having collaborated with the industry that I discovered the Medical Mafia and its machinations.

The only ones who are responsible are those who pay the bill. And that is us. Which brings me to the real purpose of this book. Namely, to shed some light on just how the medical system works, in order to better direct and focus our efforts if we wish to change it. All too often, I have seen people full of good intention devote their energy, time and money to improve a system. Only to beat their heads against a brick wall. In other words, the status quo. Quite simply, because they did not know how the system worked.

And last but not least, I would like to tell you right now that I have a weakness for fables. I will indulge in this little pleasure every once in a while. Animals and imaginary human beings relate things so well that I occasionally turn the pen (make that word-processor) over to them.

This book was conceived in the USA, modified in France, and completed in Canada. I have lived, studied and worked in the medical field in all three countries.

All three have arrived at the same setback. The same dilemma - it costs too much and one doesn't have the means to pay - despite the apparent difference of the three health systems.

I also noted that in each of the three countries, people there criticized their own system while praising that of another country without realizing that, albeit under different labels, the base was exactly the same. But then isn't grass always greener on the other side!

As if to make the point, certain Americans in authority are trying to convince the American people to adopt a Canadian-style health system. The very system that is currently helping to drive Canada to bankruptcy!

I have come to understand that:

1. We have given up trying to make sense of our own health system because it is too complicated.

2. We are all dissatisfied, no matter what the system.

3. The systems of different countries differ only in their appearance. Their very essence is the same, as well as their results: too expensive, out of control, and resulting in an increasing incidence of illness.

4. Somewhere, there must be some sort of global plan, or will, if you wish, given that the results of the systems are so much the same in all countries.

I therefore set out to find examples in these three countries, the USA, Canada and France. And to quote from works stemming from all three.

From 9 to 99

Is the medical system complicated? No. Nothing is complicated in nature. If the medical system is complicated, then it is because it has distanced itself from its very reason for being in the first place. One more reason for retrieving it and getting it back on track.

Whether you are 9 or 99, understanding your health and governing it in your own way is not a question of age. Secrecy and complexity are the tools of manipulation and the control of some by others. Transparency and simplicity are the tools of personal power. I will apply them throughout this book. If you find it simplistic, then I will have succeeded.

WHO AM I?

A doctor

I have practiced medicine in the field of phlebology (the treatment of varicose veins in the legs) for almost 20 years. Never once during this time, have I stopped asking myself questions:

- Why are certain illnesses untreatable?
- Why are some people always ill and others never?
- Why do some people die from an illness and others recover?
- Why do medical costs continue to skyrocket?
- Why are some doctors or therapists forbidden, barred from practicing, and others not?
- Why is only treatment remunerated and not prevention?
- Why are people still dying of cancer after 50 years of intensive research at astronomical cost?
- Why do governments eliminate grants to hospitals when the number of those waiting to be admitted continues to increase?
- Why do patients not know what they have. Nor why they are being operated on or what they are being treated for?
- Why are we so little informed of alternative medicines?
- Why is everyone so unhappy with the existing medical and hospital system?
- Why are there so many medical organizations and government agencies? Who's interest exactly are they protecting?

My profession was unable to provide me with any of the answers to these questions. So I gave up on hoping to learn through traditional channels. And enrolled in the school of life.

First of all with my patients. Their confidence and trust in me moved me greatly and encouraged me to always learn more so that I could better inform them. Even in areas that were not my field of specialization. They were kind enough to share their life experiences with me. I am indebted to them.

And then I went to other schools. I was out to discover all that we do not learn about medicine. Namely, **alternative medicines**. I travelled to many places, even as far as Siberia. I was determined to see for myself exactly what constitutes these different categories of medicine. I discovered a whole other parallel world medicine, which gives results that are often incredibly positive.

I also discovered, during this apprenticeship if you will, the existence and importance of that which we cannot see. The **invisible**, the **energy**. We are all vibrant bodies of energy and the frequency of these vibrations determines our state of health.

I was born an entrepreneur. Curiosity and the love of a challenge first led me to establish centres of phlebology in several towns and cities in North America. By force of circumstance, I had to grapple with the legality, business and politics of medicine. I got to rub elbows with the medical establishment.

Thanks to all these experiences, I came to understand HOW IT WORKS in medicine. Who actually controls the health system and who profits from it. My apprenticeship in the field was much different from that which I had experienced in medical school. I discovered the subtleties of the MEDICAL MAFIA and I had the answers to my questions.

In searching for an ideal medical system, I quickly realized, and it is surely no secret to anyone - that poverty is the mother of all misery - and that medical care is extremely expensive. Based on my common sense, I told myself that all one had to do was to regulate poverty in communities in order to considerably improve the finances of health. I also became very aware at this point in time that health problems were, for the most part, social and environmental problems. And that they did not require medical solutions. But rather political solutions.

Yet not only have our governments failed to regulate the social problems, they are even hacking away at all social programs that already exist. I then opened my eyes to reality. That governments have no intention whatsoever of regulating the problem. On the contrary.

A mother

As a mother of four, working for the most part with women, I realized how many of us were mistreated by my profession where misogyny reigns. I also noted the paradox that it is women who in fact are most closely involved with healthcare.

Traditionally, it is we who take care of the health of the family and it is we who consult a doctor for our husbands, our children, or for ourselves. We hold the power of the health system, but we do not exercise it. This book is therefore addressed, first and foremost, to women.

As a mother, I am convinced that the only worthwhile inheritance that I can leave my children is my contribution to the creation of a better society. A society in which they, and their children, will continue to evolve and grow.

To create, one must first of all dream. And then one must find a way to realize one's dream. **The best health, for all, at the best price.** There must be a way to achieve it. One only has to find it.

For years, I was sure that a state of health existed that was beyond the concept of "good health" that we now know, which condemns us to being ill, becoming old, and then to die.

In 1983, I put up a sign on the walls of my clinics, "HEALTH UNLIMITED". I knew it was possible, but I did not know how to arrive at it. It was not until 10 years later that I found that it could be done. I came to understand that one could achieve much more than merely maintaining a state of good health. Immortality is certainly not out of the question!

Don't worry! I do not belong to any religion, sect, secret society, or to any particular political party. My only allegiance is to myself. I am master of my thoughts, my emotions and my actions. I am my own person. A person with faith, not in external authorities, but in myself, in you, in us, in humanity. I have faith in the divinity of the human being. One only has to escape from our prison and fly. Peace, joy, health and prosperity are just behind the walls which we have unwittingly helped to erect and fortify.

To open the prison gates, I had to understand the system in order to know where I should concentrate my efforts. No treatment before first conducting a thorough diagnosis. I searched. When we search, we do discover, but not always what we would like to find - the medical system is a veritable MEDICAL MAFIA which creates sickness and kills for money and power. A rather macabre discovery.

I have assembled all the pieces of the puzzle that I have collected through-out my years of apprenticeship and I have finally reconstructed the big picture that I have dreamed of. **Unlimited health & wealth for all.**

Contrary to what all of us might like to believe, it is not the authorities, medical or political, that are going to bring about the solution. Indeed, it is they that have created the problem and it is they who seek to maintain it. We alone, as patients, as concerned citizens, can open the gate to the prison and realize our dream of health and prosperity.

I have written this book for all those of us who love life. The recipe for health is included. We only have to acquire the ingredients, mix well, and add a little dash of personal creativity. And enjoy the feast!

Bon appétit!

S.O.S. IN THE USA

The whole question of the healthcare system in the United States is currently under review. The proposed solutions do not meet the requirements of who we are. A bastardized social system for the American people. Shame! No wonder it is coming in for such close scrutiny and criticism.

The authorities are trying to present us with a rehash of other health systems from other countries. At the very time when these systems are either in the process, or on the verge, of collapsing from one day to the next.

We need to create a truly original American health system. One that is custom-designed by Americans, for Americans. And, as we are all concerned, let us all decide on the system under which we want to live. We should not leave it up to the authorities and the politicians who want to force us into a captive market and cause us to abandon our control over our health.

Control by the State under whatever banner - socialist, capitalist, conservative, liberal - is a monopoly. Controlling the money and the criteria dictating the practice of medicine, is to reduce 1,500 insurance companies to one. That is the State.

It is our money and our health. They are ours alone to control and manage. In any case, it is we who foot the bill.

As the old saying goes, " If you want something done right, then do it yourself." Certainly, we cannot do worse than the authorities have succeeded in doing to date. We can only do better. And much better at that. Quickly and without delay, let us take back control of our most prized and treasured possession, our health. And let us manage it ourselves. With common sense, fairness, and love. We will rediscover health & wealth!

AN OVERVIEW

The problem:
a medicine of sickness

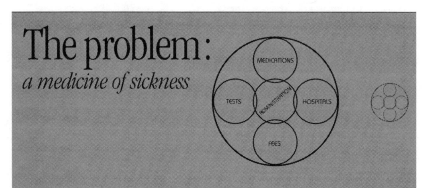

The solution:
a medicine of health

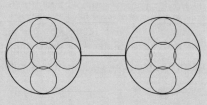

The obstacle:
the Medical Mafia

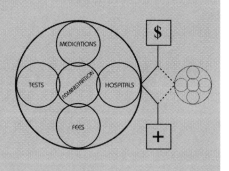

The realization:
self-health

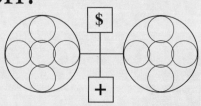

1. The medicine that is practiced is expensive and we do not have the means to continue to practice it.
2. It causes everyone to be dissatisfied. Patients and doctors alike.
3. This is true for the United States, as it is for Canada, France or, for that matter, all countries whatever their health system may be.
4. What they all have in common is a medicine of sickness called "scientific", which considers the human being to be a machine. It treats only the symptoms - the consequences of the sickness - and not the cause. It renders the patient dependent.
5. Very little money goes to health. Almost all goes to sickness. A medicine of sickness makes one ill and costs a lot.

1. If the problem is a medicine of sickness, then the solution is a medicine of health, which treats the cause of illnesses and prevents them from occurring.
2. Probably as much as 75% of the medicine of sickness is unnecessary and its cost can be avoided.
3. It is a matter of placing the emphasis on health and regulating the problems which cause sickness. These solutions have been proposed by many for a long time. In adopting them, we would be able to reduce the cost of sickness by 75% and then apply 25% of the savings to the cost of health.
4. As a result, we would have an effective "health" system at half the current cost with patients who are autonomous and responsible.
5. The solution is simple, evident and enticing. Why don't the authorities realize this? Why are they doing the very opposite?

1. The two principal actors in the system have accepted to become spectators and have relinquished their power.
   • the patients: their financial power to insurance companies, in the name of security.
   • the doctors: their medical power to institutions, in the name of protection.
2. However, security and protection are illusions. Belief in them, in effect, means that the actors have become spectators, prisoners of a system of sickness which costs them dearly and which makes them ill.
3. If both patients and doctors are dissatisfied, someone else out there must be happy that such a medical system is being perpetuated and that it is being "installed" around the world.
4. Who then created the system and is keeping it in place? Surely those that profit from it. It is the industry that reaps large profits and it is the industry that is keeping the establishment (established medicine) in power which, in turn, keeps patients and doctors captives of a system of sickness.
5. Officially, we are told that the system is at the service of the patient. But, in practice, the system is at the service of the industry which pulls the strings and maintains a system of sickness for its own profit. That is the MEDICAL MAFIA.

1. The two principal actors in the system take back their respective power:
   • the patients: their financial power
   • the doctors: their medical power
2. The only one who has the ultimate power to change the system is the patient, the very reason for being of the system. The patients will take back their power over health and exercise their sovereignty. The doctors recognize the sovereignty of the patients and help them to exercise it. That is self-health.
3. There will follow a patient-doctor-therapist partnership based on the collaboration between equal partners in health. It is the way to transform the present medical system.
4. Such partnerships will extend to one and all. And this will be true universal healthcare.
5. Finally, we will realize HEALTH & WEALTH FOR ALL.

The problem:
a medicine of sickness

THREE COUNTRIES, THREE SYSTEMS

Over the years, I have divided my time between the United States, Canada and France. In each of these countries, I have heard, and still hear today, the same refrain: "The health system costs too much and we just do not have the means to continue with it". And yet, these three countries all have a different form of health system.

- The United States has a health system that is very little socialized. **Medicare** with access limited to those 65 and over. **Medicaid** with limited access to those really in need. The majority of the population is covered by private insurance, individual or group, paid for in large part by their employers. A large percentage of the population (estimated to be close to 40 million) has no health insurance whatsoever.

- Canada has a health system that is socialized. **Healthcare** insurance with universal access and limited coverage.

- France has a health system that is very socialized. **Social Security** (SECU) with universal access and extensive coverage.

Deterioration and dissatisfaction

In addition to sky-rocketing costs, the state of health is deteriorating before our very eyes. Cancer, AIDS and auto-immune illnesses, degenerative illnesses such as Alzheimer's disease, each one more bizarre than the other, take their daily toll. And we are powerless to stop them. They are devastating our population and our wallets.

Moreover, dissatisfaction reigns. So what is the common cause of these three health systems that they all suffer from the same symptoms?

STUDY OF A SYSTEM

A system is an arranged order of elements. This entails:
- several elements
- disposed in a certain order
- to make a whole

We must therefore:
- identify the elements
- find the order that governs them
- determine the desired result

Whether it involves a simple system or a complex one, the principles are always the same. Whether it be:
- a human being
- society
- health
- planet Earth

All have an identical structure and order. They suffer from the same illnesses and require the same treatments. One only has to study one in order to understand them all. I would like to explore with you that of the human being.

What is a human being?

It is a BEING which has a human body. We are in the presence of a duality. To be and to have. This duality finds itself:

- either in opposition. That is war, illness, disorder.
- or in harmony. That is peace, health, order.

One only has to find the right frequency and get on the right "wavelength" for all to go well. It is as simple as that.

The quest for Truth

For millennia, we have sought to know:

1. who we are.
2. where we come from.
3. where we are going.
4. what we are doing on Earth.

These questions often remain unanswered or receive an answer with a question mark tagged on. Yet one cannot approach the subject of the health of a human being without first posing these questions. It is in all modesty that I have outlined some tentative answers. And yet the TRUTH is there. Right at our fingertips, but so difficult to grasp.

My research and questioning have led me to arrive at certain observations and conclusions that are far different from those of my medical, philosophical and religious teachings. In the pages that follow, I will share with you the summary of my extra-curricular apprenticeship. It is the truth as I know it. And it is only of value to me. But perhaps it will encourage you in your quest for your own truth. That is all that it can do for you.

A body, a soul, a spirit

To the question: who are we? The answer is: a body, a soul, and a spirit.

We often come across these three words, but with different meanings, explanations and functions. I resume here that which I have understood and while incomplete, hopefully, it will help you to also understand how our system works. To learn why it is sometimes out of balance. And to discover how we can make it work in perfect harmony.

BODY		SOUL	SPIRIT
visible structure	invisible envelopes	conscience	I Am
physical	emotions/thoughts	intention	God/Goddess
visible	invisible	invisible	invisible
mortal	mortal	immortal	eternal
very low vibrations	low vibrations	high vibrations	very high vibrations
procreative energy		co-creative energy	creative energy
personality		individuality	divinity
external power		internal power	all powerful

WHO IS AT THE SERVICE OF WHOM?

MATTER	C H O I C E ?	SPIRIT
appearance		essence
creature		creator
shadow		light
illusion		reality
finite		infinite
sickness/death		health/life
vehicle		traveller
TO HAVE		**TO BE**

BODY		SOUL	SPIRIT
THE VISIBLE PHYSICAL BODY which we can all see because its vibrations are low. It is our body in flesh and bone. It is touchable and measurable. It is easy to understand. It functions by physical and chemical reactions based on the physics of Newton. All is explicable and predictable. Since the physical body also vibrates, it may be influenced by emotions and thoughts which control its hormonal and nervous systems. Its state of health depends entirely upon that of invisible bodies.	**THE INVISIBLE BODIES.** They envelop the visible body. They are four in number: 1) the **ethereal** body, molded on the physical body. 2) the **emotional** body, the seat of emotions. 3) the **mental** body, the seat of thoughts. 4) the **spiritual** body, assures relations with others and the external world. Few people can see these bodies because their vibrations are already too rapid for the naked eye. But we know from experience that our morale influences our physical being. Positive thoughts and emotions assure health, while certain beliefs and fear lead to sickness.	The soul is the link which joins the Light Source (Cosmos) to the Earth. It captains the journey of the spirit in matter. It knows from where it comes and where it is going. It has a charted map and it knows the itinerary. If it remains true to the divine plan, its intentions are also true. Then all goes well. It is order and health. If it submits to external thought pressures (beliefs) and emotions (fear), it loses itself in matter. It is disorder and sickness. The vibrations of the soul are higher than those of the bodies. Its influence on them is direct and rapid.	The spirit is the Light in all of us, emanating from the Source. The spirit is the very essence, the substance, the reason for being of a human being. No spirit, no matter. It exists unto itself. It comes to travel on earth and takes a vehicle, the body. The spirit is the original, the body the copy. The spirit is eternal. The body lasts only the duration of the journey. It is temporary and mortal. The spirit is everywhere. It is Light, the highest vibration of all. It heals all others. It is perfect. It is God/Goddess fused together. It is androgenous. It is divine. Therefore, the human being is of divine nature. It is all-powerful, health, life. It cannot be sick. It is unlimited health.

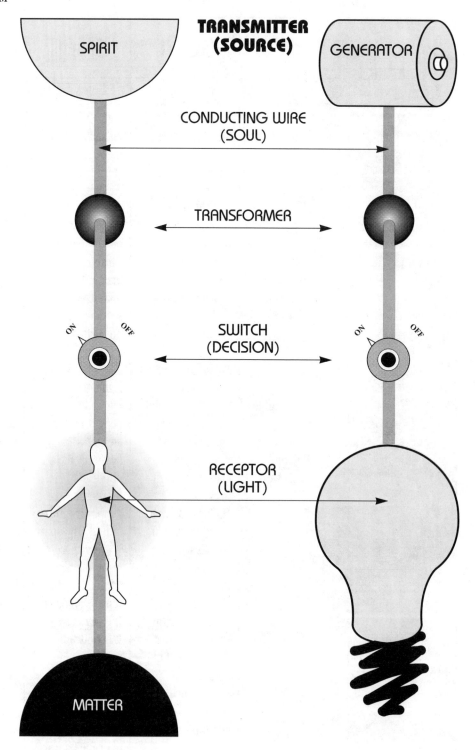

TRANSMITTER
(SOURCE)

SPIRIT

GENERATOR

CONDUCTING WIRE
(SOUL)

TRANSFORMER

ON   OFF   SWITCH   ON   OFF
               (DECISION)

RECEPTOR
(LIGHT)

MATTER

An electrical system

We can compare our energy system to an electrical system.

- Electricity comes from the Light Source, creative, cosmic.
- It is transmitted along a wire, along which there are many relays and transformers to reduce the intensity and protect matter. However, by increasing the frequency of matter, we reduce the need for relays and transformers. We are thus able to get more in tune with our Source.
- The current can only pass when the switch is ON.
- The Light is captured by a receptor which lights up.
- It in turn illuminates the organism.

It is important to note that one must take the decision to turn the switch ON in order for the electricity to pass. Without that decision, there is no light. One remains in the dark.

The enigmatic soul

"In all honesty", we often say that when we listen to our innermost selves. And saying that, we know that we are in accord with ourselves. What exactly do we mean by that? To be in accord means that one is on the same wavelength, the same frequency. As whom, as what? We know that it is our spirit, our Energy, that nourishes each and every one of our cells. The music flows. We feel good with ourselves. There is peace. When there is discord between our body and our spirit, there is no harmony or accord, but rather dissension. We are strung-out and out of sync. It is disorder, suffering, sickness.

What is the soul?

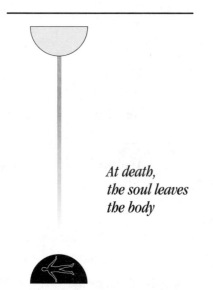

At death, the soul leaves the body

It is the wire along which flows the electricity from the power station. It transmits electricity from that station to the light bulb. It transmits Vital Energy from the Source to every cell in the body, without which they die.

"He gave up his soul at 2:35," is the often-heard saying when describing the exact moment when a person dies. It is the exact time when the soul departs its body.

The soul is the energizing spinal column of the entire body. It is to the invisible body what the vertebral column is to the visible body. Its state cannot be measured by instruments, but it can be perceived. There are several common expressions that describe it well.

WORDS THAT DESCRIBE
THE STATE OF THE SOUL

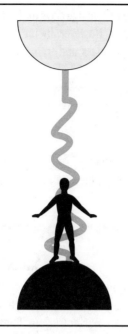

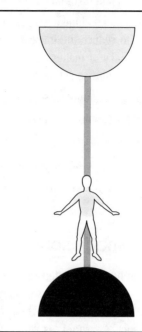

Sick soul:	**Healthy soul:**
• orchestra conductor controlled: submissive	• orchestra conductor is in control: sovereign
• human being dragged down	• human being rises

Petty	Generous
Growels	Dignified
Closed	Open
Cowers	Stands tall
Disconnected	Tuned in
Stoops	Stands up
Broken	Confident
Devious	Direct
Complicated	Uncomplicated
Twisted	Straight
Soft	Firm
Fragile	Solid as a rock

What does the soul do?

It brings life and health to the organism. It is the orchestra conductor. It arranges and directs the score for every musician (visible and invisible bodies) so that they play in harmony with the tune (spirit). But still, we have to listen.

The health of the system, or of our organism, depends upon the efficiency of the orchestra conductor: the **conscience.**

- If the orchestra conductor is not alert or asleep, it is cacophony. Each body plays its part of the composition at its own frequency or rhythm.
- If the orchestra conductor is alert and awake, it is a sheer delight. Each body plays the same melody in harmony with the frequency of the others.

The more awakened the state of consciousness, the healthier the bodies.

What can lull the consciousness to sleep? Matter, the denser it is, the lower the vibrations, and the less the soul can be heard.

1. The sleeping pill of the physical body is **intoxication**. It distorts the conscience by alcohol, noise, work, gambling, success, sex, consumption, and whatever else comes into play.

2. The sleeping pill of the emotional body is **fear**. The fear of not HAVING that which one wants, or fear of LOSING that which one already HAS. It cripples the consciousness. It buries one alive in a coffin of ice.

3. The third sleeping pill, that of the mental body, is **belief.** Belief in preconceived ideas, rather than conceiving them for oneself from one's soul, which knows all. It imprisons the conscience.

4. Even if the consciousness is awake, it can be fooled. One can charm and so captivate it that even though we hear it, it does not worry us, or become a pain in the side. One buys its silence. It is **corruption**. One sells one soul for material gain. Prestige, money, power. After all, it was not only Faust who sold his soul to the devil. We all do it every day.

Intoxication, fear, belief and corruption all have the same consequence. The submission of the soul to the body. The natural order is thrown into a state of confusion. From here grows disorder, sickness, war, misery, death. They sabotage our individual health, that of our systems, that of our society.

THE HEALTH OF THE SOUL DETERMINES THE HEALTH OF THE BODIES

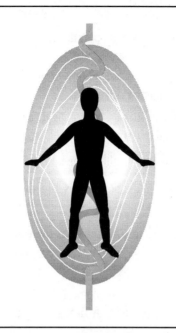 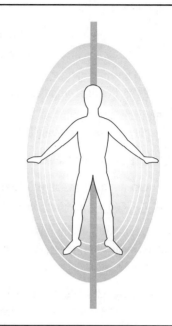

sickness	**health**
• orchestra conductor unaware, unalert • bodies are heavy, obscure.	• orchestra conductor awake: alert and conscious • bodies are light and luminous.
The more the soul is twisted, the poorer it transmits the Source's Light.	The truer the soul, the better it transmits the Source's Light.
The lower the vibrations of the soul.	The higher the vibrations of the soul.
The lower the level of consciousness.	The higher the level of consciousness.
The more thoughts and emotions dominate.	The more it controls and facilitates the passage of Light.
The more the bodies lower their vibrations.	The more the bodies raise the level of their vibrations.
The greater the disharmony with the Source's Light.	The more they harmonize with the Source's Light.
The heavier and more obscure the bodies.	The more the bodies are light and luminous.

Four dimensions, four worlds

Two bodies (one visible and one invisible), a soul, and a spirit. That makes four. Four dimensions *(Barbara Brennan)* or four worlds *(Janine Fontaine)*. These four worlds, while different, all have points in common.

They all vibrate

Even the physical body vibrates. It is made up of vibrations with such low frequencies that we refer to them as heavy. That is why we can see it with the naked eye. The three other worlds (invisible body, soul, spirit) have vibrations with ever-increasing frequencies and we refer to them as light or subtle. This is why we cannot see them. For example, the eagle, when it flies, we see the flapping of its majestic wings at a slow frequency, even when it is flying at full speed. The humming-bird, on the other hand, beats its wings at such a rapid frequency that they cannot be seen.

The highest, or lightest, vibratory frequency is that of the spirit, the Source of all vibrations. It is the Light which progressively passes through the other three dimensions or worlds to be subsequently found in each of even the tiniest particles in our physical body. The easier it passes through these, the higher it raises their vibratory frequencies during its passage. As a result, they are in good health. And we, in turn, become healthier.

They are all describable

We cannot see, nor can we touch, the vibrations because they are not in material form. It is not because we cannot see or measure them, however, that they do not exist. It is because our capacity for extrasensory perception is atrophied or asleep. It is also because our instruments for measurement are simply not up to the task. Yet some people have the ability - innate or acquired - to perceive or feel the vibrations of the bodies or soul, to the point of being able to describe and quantify them. Several books have been written telling us about the subtle (invisible) components of the human being. They provide us with their description, their functioning, their sicknesses, their treatments. I refer you to two of these authors.

- In France, *Janine Fontaine*, a Doctor of cardiology and anesthesiology, has developed an extraordinary sensibility which enables her to evaluate the state of subtle (invisible) bodies. Since 1977, she has practiced a form of energetic medicine. She has written several books in which she describes in detail the energetic body and the physical rules which govern it.

- In the USA, *Barbara Brennan*, a scientist and therapist, has developed an extraordinary clairvoyance which enables her to "see" the subtle dimensions of the human being. She shares the result of her research, describes her practice as a healer, and her teachings, in two well-illustrated books. In them, she also teaches us to use our inner power of healing.

SEE to BELIEVE
or
BELIEVE to SEE

They are all interdependent

Whatever happens in one of the worlds affects the others. When one is affected by a problem, so too are the others. This interdependence follows a natural order. The worlds influence one another, starting from the lightest vibrations to the heaviest. That is to say, from the spirit to the soul, then to the invisible body and, finally, to the visible physical body. When sickness occurs in the physical body, it has already occurred in first the soul and then the invisible body. The spirit, however, is never sick. It is the source of healing for the bodies. It IS health. As for the soul, it transmits health. For its part, the physical body manifests health.

Sickness never begins in the physical body, unless it stems from some kind of accident. In general, health begins to deteriorate in the soul whose alteration immediately affects the invisible body. However, the attack on the invisible body can take years to physically manifest itself. This is to say that:

- one doesn't catch an illness. Rather one develops illness and sometimes it takes years before becoming evident and apparent.
- one can diagnose eventual illnesses by evaluating the state of health of the invisible body.
- one can therefore prevent illnesses by treating the invisible body before the sickness takes hold.
- it is better to treat the sickness by respecting the order of its appearance. In other words, treating the most subtle body and working towards the least subtle. In this way, it is possible that one does not have to work on the physical body at all, contrary to what we usually do. The healing of the invisible body will automatically lead to that of the physical body, providing that there is no real physical emergency involved, which goes without saying.

They all follow the Universal Law

The **Universal Law** is the order which rules the Universe. It is the divine cosmic order, which causes events to arrive at the right time and in the right place. It is the order which governs all natural functions of our organism and those of all organisms. It is called the **Natural Order.**

This order is transmitted even into our cells, ensuring that they function well. When they are disturbed, the opposite is true. For then comes disorder, sickness and death.

The **Universal Law** is cosmic, divine, and comes from the lightest vibrations of all. It therefore governs the:

PRIORITY OF THE SPIRIT OVER MATTER

to maintain our individual good health, that of society, and that of Planet Earth.

A journey on planet Earth

To the question, what are we doing here? The answer is, a journey on planet EARTH. The word journey has two implications:

- a goal, a 'raison d'être' or reason for being
- a beginning and an end

We are therefore in passage, in a place which is not ours, and where we come as visitors.

Why do we come on Earth?

I ask myself why would we, as a spirit/traveller, who is light and free, want to burden ourselves with a body/vehicle to make a journey on a planet plagued with disasters, suffering, wars, violence, misery, sickness, and death?

- either we are masochistic. In which case we should feel fulfilled;
- or we want to become richer. In which case we are going to be deceived. Nobody, to my knowledge, has ever left with their worldly possessions. They are far too heavy.
- or we want to learn something. Perhaps to triumph over matter.

And if it is only to fly faster and higher? Then why not? Jonathan Livingstone Seagull succeeded! You may have asked yourself why millions of people worldwide have read a story of a bird which tried to fly a little higher every day. What could be more insignificant? Unless this bird succeeded in realizing our secret dream!

For that is the challenge that this planet presents. To come and play in the material world in order to learn how to transcend it. Unfortunately, we forget the 'raison d'être' of our journey and we allow ourselves to become suffocated and smothered by this very matter that we wish to transcend.

To my patients who are concerned about their physical appearance, I ask them what they came to do on Earth. When they do not know, I tell them this little story.

Once upon a time, a woman wanted to visit the California wine country. She decided to take a trip for a month.

She flew to California, rented a car which met her needs, and set off. On the highway, she saw billboards advertising cars that were faster than hers. So she stopped at a car rental garage and changed hers for another model. And she set off again. Rolling along, she saw signs pointing to the ski slopes. She followed the arrows. Before she knew it, her car broke down in snow right up to the axles. She had to spend several days at the garage while they changed the oil to a winter grade and installed winter tires. And set off again.

Still rolling along, she saw other billboards advertising red cars. Hers was white. She turned off into a car bodyshop and had it painted red.

But time ran out when, suddenly, she remembered that she had come to California to visit the vineyards. Unfortunately, she had spent all her time in garages. And now it was time to leave.

She realized that our body is only a rented vehicle!

Our soul knows...we know that:

1. Our body is leased to make our journey. We chose it to meet our apprenticeship needs. Love it as it is and stop trying to make it fit the standards established by others.

2. Human nature is good. It is of divine spirit. Each entity on Earth is of identical nature, for it is issued from the same Source, the same origin. We are all members of the same family, equal brothers and sisters.

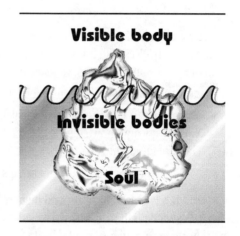

3. Like the iceberg, the most important part is not visible. Similarly, in human beings, it is the soul which enables the body to exist.

4. Divine entities, which we are, are capable of everything. They can therefore cure themselves. "Spontaneous remissions" are normal. Sickness and death are not.

5. Laws of the material world are but illusions. They have no power over the cosmic reality. To submit to them is to renounce our freedom and reduce ourselves to slavery.

6. It is our soul which directs the show. The awakened state and alertness of our orchestra conductor (consciousness) determines the vibratory frequency of our body. The higher it is, the more we are in harmony with the Source's Light, the more we are in good health.

That which applies to human beings also applies to every structured organism or system. Whether it be:

- a person, an animal, or thing
- a system: medical, economic, political
- a society: village, region, country
- a planet: Earth

one always finds duality

MATTER - SPIRIT
BODY - SOUL

Each system is confronted with the same fundamental question:

WHO IS AT THE SERVICE OF WHOM?

"WHO IS AT THE SERVICE OF WHOM?"

THE FUNDAMENTAL QUESTION

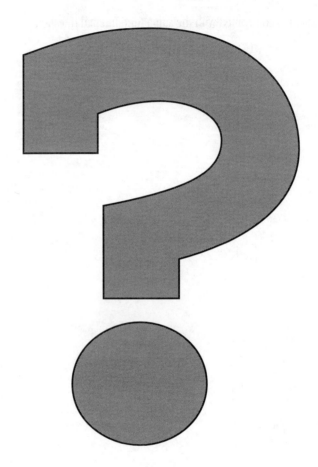

The spirit at the service of matter,
or
matter at the service of the spirit.

The fundamental question

Is the traveler at the service of the vehicle, or the vehicle at the service of the traveler? That is the fundamental question which underlies the thought process throughout this book. It is for each of us to answer in our own way.

Only we have the capability of choosing. This capability is found in the SOUL, the seat of conscience and of will. Depending upon our level of consciousness, we will take the decision either to give matter priority over the spirit, or the spirit over matter.

Right now, we are living in a materialistic world in which matter has priority over spirit, and in which, as a result, **the spirit is at the service of matter.** Matter, we know, is made up of heavy and very low vibrations. It is limited in time and space and leads to suffering, illness, aging and death.

But unlike the animals we have, thanks to our freedom of choice, the possibility of changing this materialistic priority into a spiritual priority in which, as a result, **matter will be at the service of the spirit.** We will come to know joy, health, youth, and eternity.

It is up to us to choose!

MATTER	SPIRIT
vehicle	traveler
appearance	essence
illusion	reality
unconsciousness/ unawareness	consciousness/ awareness
external god	internal God/Goddess
fear/beliefs	love
slave	master
TO HAVE	**TO BE**

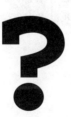

A MEDICINE OF SICKNESS

The systems that we describe as ones of health are, in fact, systems of sickness. There is simply no other word for it. We practice a **medicine of sickness** which:

- is only concerned with sickness, not health;
- recognizes only the existence of the body;
- treats only the symptoms, not the cause;
- keeps the patient in the dark and dependent;
- encourages consumption.

Sickness YES, Health NO

Nothing is allocated for health in health insurance rates. Only sickness is refundable. When doctors find nothing abnormal, they almost have to forge a diagnosis for the insurance. Try to imagine the following scene. You show up at your doctor's office and announce that you want to improve your state of health. And that you want his or her help to achieve this. The response may well be: **"Health? We don't treat health."** If you are lucky enough to be a smoker, even just a few a day, you can be sure that you are in for a sermon. If not, you will leave empty handed. I advise you not to insist too much because, if you do, you may be diagnosed as obsessive and entered into the computer as a psychiatric case. And then you will be given a prescription for some pills to calm your nerves.

This is not done out of ill will, but out of ignorance. Over the years, we doctors have been taught sickness, but never health. The definition of health is the absence of sickness. If you are not ill, you are automatically in good health and therefore you don't need us.

Impossible health

Rates determine the revenue of doctors. Yet the visit, that is to say the regular contact between doctor and patient, is an act that is most poorly remunerated. And yet it is the act that is the most important. Conscientious doctors who do take the time, be it half-an-hour to an hour per patient, are barely able to cover their operating costs. Rates are set by governments and insurance companies alike so that they force doctors to limit time they spend with their patients to a minimum.

Doctors, therefore, replace talking with their patients, doing detailed examinations, giving advice and encouragement, by ordering tests, prescribing medications, or recommending surgical interventions.

Treating symptoms, normalizing the figures

A symptom is a physical manifestation of a problem far deeper than that which we can see. Our organism is a marvelous machine which is constantly adjusting to all conditions that it is subjected to, without ever saying a word. It is only when it is overloaded that it signals us by displaying certain symptoms. **Symptoms are the language of the body**. What an opportunity!

Thus, fever is the manifestation of the body that defends itself against an attack or aggression. It is a sign of health. Don't try and make it normal. Unfortunately, the medicine of sickness doesn't listen! It is designed to silence the symptoms, such as pain, tiredness, discomfort, to make the signs, such as fever, swelling and inflammation, a tumor, disappear, to re-establish the figures relating to cholesterol, sugar, calcium, to "normalize" behaviour in instances of depression, anxiety, and the like.

A symptom, like the tip of an iceberg, is desirable. It does us a favour. It tells us that something much bigger is amiss beneath the surface. Treating the symptoms is just like cutting off the part of the iceberg that is showing above the surface. No wonder we're surprised when our boat then crashes into it and sinks.

Not only are we doing a disservice to our body by treating the symptom, but we are making ourselves even sicker with all the medicines and drugs that we use to treat. And that's not even talking about surgery. Every time this happens, we are screwing up the body even more at a time when it is already having problems staying afloat. We are destroying our health. We are making ourselves ill. Why do doctors do it? Because that's what's taught: illness, and, not to forget, respect for scientific dogma.

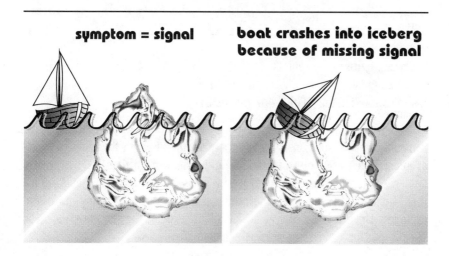

symptom = signal

boat crashes into iceberg because of missing signal

Ignoring the problem

It is not because we cannot see the problem that it does not exist. Problems are always "hidden". We must search them out. But do we?

We are products of a materialistic civilization and we want our physical problems (symptoms and signs) remedied quickly. That is what we expect from a doctor and that is what we receive. Moreover, medicine is also materialistic in its conception. In the name of the holier-than-thou Science, it recognizes only matter which it can see, touch and measure. Nothing else seems to exist.

To scientific medicine, a person is no more than a visible physical body.

- without thoughts or emotions (invisible bodies)
- without a conscience (soul)

In addition, it denies the very essence of a human being, the spirit. Yet the sickness always travels up from the "depths" before it shows itself on the surface.

VISIBLE tip	ICEBERG	result of problem
INVISIBLE bodies		problem
base: SOUL		cause of problem

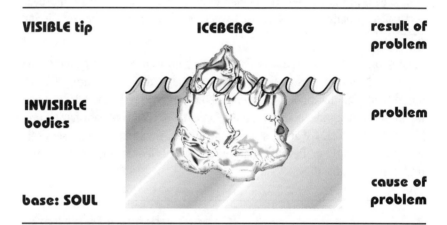

Sickness **begins** in the soul: the CAUSE
It **settles** in the invisible bodies: the PROBLEM
It **shows itself** in the visible body: the RESULT

Not correcting the problem is expensive, because it keeps manifesting itself. Sometimes in the same guise, sometimes in another. But it is the same "hidden" problem which cries out a warning... and... help! Each time, it cries a little louder, each time, we respond to it with stronger and stronger medications. Right up until the day when the body simply cannot take it any more and explodes. Then, it is an emergency situation. Hospital. Surgery. Test after test. The octopus has us in its tentacles. The nightmare begins.

Causing illnesses

They are known as iatrogenic illnesses. They are generated by the medical system. They are extremely well described by Ivan Illich in his book entitled, ***Medical Nemesis - The Expropriation of Health.***

Not content with removing the patients' awareness and refusing the true meaning of the pain and illness, medicine makes them even more ill. I can't help but think of the vaccines which wipe out the defense systems of children. Sometimes as many as 20 are administered before they even start school. And then one wonders why they suffer repeatedly from otitis (which one treats with antibiotics) and later in life, from allergies, cancers, multiple sclerosis, AIDS, etc. The list of illnesses is long in an immune-depressed population.

It is interesting to note that vaccines only appeared for the first time after the major epidemics had almost disappeared naturally, by themselves. But the dangers of vaccine are never mentioned or reported, unless they result in a strong reaction right after the vaccination.

A third of all people admitted to hospitals are there because of the negative effects of medications. 700,000 Americans die each year of secondary effects from medications!

Medical Nemesis
Ivan Illich

Creating illnesses

In the name of **prevention**, one attacks, mutilates, destroys. And we ruin ourselves financially in the process. Take pregnancy, for example. What could be more normal? Our ancestors were having babies that were just as healthy and as normal as ours, and in even larger numbers, without ever visiting a doctor.

But not any more. In the name of prevention, or perhaps that the baby will be malformed, or I know not what, the mother becomes a pawn on the chessboard of the medical system. Not to know how SHE is. But to see if the baby is normal. That is to say, that the baby meets all the statistical norms.

Sometimes, the mother is made to undergo echograms. If only the baby could speak! Then if her weight should happen to increase, the doctor reprimands and scares her. From now on, she is worried. But it gets worse if any one parameter does not fit the norm or is in doubt.

Then a hellish investigation begins. If the baby is not following its pre-determined schedule, birth is induced, or a caesarean ordered. And to avoid any future problems, the mother will invariably have a caesarean from now on. For so-called normal births, it is routine to have an episiotomy. That is to say, a large deep cut in the vagina so as to prevent lacerations.

Every **normal** stage in a woman's life is treated as an illness. This is true of menstruation and PMS. Also menopause, for which one automatically prescribes hormones in order to avoid the so-called complications. And as for mammograms to prevent breast cancer, this is not prevention. It is only a detection device to treat it earlier. The tests are often wrong. But the treatment continues

Premenstrual syndrome (PMS) has just been classified as a psychiatric illness in the DMS, the bible of diagnostics. To be a woman is now synonymous with being crazy!

all the same. I am going to stop listing examples of how women's bodies are mutilated and exploited, the list is simply too long!

It is not only women, however. Children who do not fit the accepted pattern are also subjected to medication. A child who is rebellious or doesn't fit into the standardized statistical norm is considered to be "hyperactive" and is made to take medication for a fictitious illness.

All this is what is called **medicalization of society.** It is very well explained by Joel Lexchin in his book, ***The Real Pushers - A Critical Analysis of the Canadian Drug Industry.*** Also by Lynn Payer in her recent book, ***Disease-Mongers. How doctors, drug companies and insurers are making you feel sick.***

Pharmaceutical companies show us, and with figures to back it up, that the cost of medications does not exceed 5% of total health costs. And that a large part of their budgets goes to research. They conveniently forget to tell us that their advertising and promotional budget is two to three times greater than their research budget. Also that their research is focused on existing profitable products and not new ones, which certain illnesses are greatly in need of. They are also not the ones who will tell us that medication is the cause of many illnesses, a third of the cost of hospitilizations, and of many deaths.

Disease-Mongers
Lynn Payer

A LITTLE HISTORY

*"Those who cannot remember their history
are condemned to repeat it"*

Medicine that we practice today is one of sickness. Has it always been this way?

Witches Midwives and Nurses
Barbara Enrenreich Deirdre English

No. As the vast majority of problems are minor and are related to the emotions, they do not require extraordinary medical intervention. Rather, the individual needs to be listened to, advised, and reassured. In addition, it is women who tend to look after the family's health and who consult a doctor on behalf of their children and even their husbands. Health has always been the concern of women.

Taking "care" of someone is essentially a feminine profession. It requires feeling, intuition, insight, observation, compassion, devotion, love and wisdom. These qualities are all inherent to the feminine principle, which is more developed in women, children, the elderly, the humble, and those gifted with extra-sensory powers. This is why healthcare was essentially provided by women. Mothers of families and grandmothers with their lists of remedies. Nurses. Also by midwives, healers, phytotherapists, etc. They practiced an empirical medicine, based on experience and common sense. Health did not cost a lot and all poor had access to it. The people called them wise people. The authorities treated them as witches and charlatans.

Because the Church, then all-powerful, considered sickness to be a punishment from God for the sins that one had committed, it found sickness, suffering and death to be salutary and beneficial. And it therefore discouraged the practice of medicine. It was not until the 13th century that the Church accepted that medicine be practiced. Medical schools were born in the universities. From which women were excluded.

And so appeared official medicine, dominated by men. It was strictly controlled by the Church, which imposed its doctrines upon it. Medicine recognized by the authorities was based on superstition. It was practiced by men and served the rich. Very early on, the authorities forbade anyone who did not have a diploma to practice medicine.

The arrival of men on the medical scene sounded the beginning of the elimination of the medicine practiced by women. That which was practical, effective, and inexpensive.

So why do we now practice almost exclusively a medicine of sickness? And which costs us a fortune?

The answer is, the elimination of health practitioners by the authorities to serve their own interests. Whether it be the religious laws of the Inquisition in the Middle Ages or the medical laws of our own century, the result is always the same. A minority of privileged people make laws to dominate and exploit the majority, particularly those most in need in our society. It is history merely repeating itself.

Malleus Maleficarum

From 1257 to 1816. The Inquisition tortured and burned millions of innocent people. They were accused of heresy towards religious dogma. Of witchcraft. They were judged without due trial, in secret, under the terror of torture. If they "confessed", they were declared guilty of witchcraft. If they did not "confess", they were then found guilty of heresy. Then they were burned at the stake. Nobody could escape. Some historians have estimated that in three centuries, close to nine million "witches" were exterminated. Some 80% of them were women and children.

Women were also raped while they were being tortured. All their worldly goods were confiscated from the very moment they were accused, before even being brought to trial. For nobody was spared. Their children and families were dispossessed. Even the dead were dug up and their bones burned.

Every woman who was not married, and who displayed an unusual characteristic, or a particular feature or trait, and that even included having red hair, could be accused of witchcraft. The authorities declared it as heresy if one did not consider witches to be dangerous.

The Manual of the Inquisition, the Malleus Maleficarum (the Mallet of Witches) stipulated that the accused witch had to be "often and frequently exposed to torture." This reign of terror would last five centuries. And it received the blessing of Church and State alike.

Heresy is an idea, theory or practice which goes against the opinions and dogma of the authorities.

Why the terror? To dominate and exploit the population. To impose a religion that the population did not want. And to enrich the dignitaries (the religious authorities) and their accomplices (the inquisitors). These, incidentally, enjoyed special privileges. They were above the law.

Why women? To eliminate the feminine principle. Because they had the natural leadership role in the community, women threatened the power of the authorities. They took care of health and men learned with them. They passed on traditions from one generation to the next. Elderly women solved disputes and arguments with dignity and wisdom. They had a natural power. They were powerful. They represented the sovereignty of the feminine principle with values of conservation, protection, helping one another, sharing. They, in turn, made the majority of the population powerful.

Although women were the prime target, it did not matter whether you were a man or woman. Anyone who had a brain represented a threat to the richness and power of the privileged minority. Therefore, they had to be eliminated. In order to do this, one declared them witches.

From the beginning of time, the authorities, whether they be aristocratic, religious, or financial, have fought to maintain their patriarchal domination and exploitation. It is still true today.

Flexner Report

From 1910 to 1925. Thanks to rules established in the **Flexner Report**, the *American Medical Association* (AMA) and the *Association of American Medical Colleges* (AMC) would eliminate the vast majority of natural therapists. In the name of science and the quality of the practice of medicine, demands are made on medical schools to adopt the recommendations of the **Flexner Report**. It is the reign of terror in the medical world. The schools have to take the new scientific orientation imposed by the latter and its financial backers, or they will be made to close their doors.

Yet at this time, there were twice as many practitioners of alternative medicine than there were of orthodox medicine (allopathic). Homeopathy, phytotherapy, manipulative medicines such as osteopathy and massage were then taught. Medical reform eliminated them all. The number of medical schools was slashed from 650 to 50. As was the number of students, from 7,500 to 2,500. The future of health fell into the hands of the elite male rich. Medicine became a service tool of high finance. The Carnegie and Rockefeller Foundations had financed the Report and its application. **The world of finance took over control of medicine which it has exploited ever since,** with the disastrous results that are now evident.

Their accomplices are the powerful "expert" doctors who enjoy such privileges as power, money and prestige. It is a North-American monopoly. Any attempt to deviate from their "ways" or practice alternative medicine is severely reprimanded. In the name of the well-being of the population, one accuses these practitioners of heresy. Of being charlatans. And they are subject to harassment and intimidation, the loss of their right to practice and being hounded to the letter of the law. The Inquisition is alive and well today.

Declaration of Alma Ata

In 1977. The **Declaration of Alma Ata** gave to the World Health Organization (W.H.O.) the means to extend the Flexner Report not only in North America, but throughout the entire world. Again, in the name of health and the well-being of the populations of the world, and in respect of the right of "health for all", international criteria and rules were established for practicing medicine. Control of health, therefore, was transferred from national governments to a world government. A world government that is non-elected. And of which its "Surgeon General" in charge of health is the W.H.O.

> **"Competition is a sin"**
> J.D. Rockefeller

And what does the right to health mean? It means **the right to medicalization**. It opens the doors wide to a medicine of **global** sickness, whether we want it or not. Vaccinations and medications are imposed on people around the world. And then we are amazed that they are dying of AIDS.

This global manipulation is extremely subtle. Just when our country's population is beginning to become aware of the industry's control over health and government corruption, and is demanding change, the world authorities arrive like a knight in shining armor in the name of the well-being of people everywhere. And with our consent. We are totally mystified. For who would doubt the honourable intentions of the W.H.O.

> **"We shall have a world government, whether or not you like it - by conquest or consent."**
> James Warburg, banker, CFR member, testifying before the US Senate, in 1950.

But who actually controls that the W.H.O.? That is the question. And also the answer. The United Nations (U.N.), the political arm of world financiers, that includes those who backed the Flexner Report and its application. More and more subtly, the medical and political authorities are robbing us of what is ours, as well as our rights. They establish the rules and make the laws that exploit us. It is a regime of medical terror. It is a world monopoly. Beware those who oppose it. The witch-hunt continues, but now on a global scale!

MALLEUS MALEFICARUM	FLEXNER REPORT	ALMA ATA
Europe	North America	The World
Middle Ages	1910	1977

HOW MUCH DOES IT COST?

Using generally accepted ballpark figures, what does it cost per person every year to have the right to be sick?

- In the United States: $3,000.
- In Canada and France: $2,000.

We can see that the costs are higher in the United States for results obtained in terms of life expectancy, infant mortality that are equivalent, and perhaps even less, than in the two other countries. Rather than trying to analyze or justify figures, suffice it to say that the systems in all three countries are totally out of whack.

A doctor who is very highly placed in France's health insurance hierarchy (SECU) told me in confidence with a profound feeling of helplessness: **"The system is drifting aimlessly"**. The Canadian and French governments are cutting back everywhere and are regularly reducing services. Despite that, their health systems are still in a state of disarray. The American system is no worse. It is just more expensive. This doesn't make the Canadian and French systems any better.

In the United States, close to nine-hundred-and-forty-billion dollars ($940,000,000,000) was spent in 1993. This adds up to much more than $3,000 per person. But let's be conservative so that it is easier to do the adding up. And don't forget that we are talking about ballpark figures. We will see later just what these figures represent in our day-to-day lives. And how they affect our life as a whole.

At the national level

The American health budget is expected to shortly reach the trillion dollar mark ($1,000,000,000,000). What do all these zeros mean? I don't know if you are like me, but after a certain number of zeros, I'm lost. When figures reach a certain level, they lose all their meaning. I have therefore tried to interpret them in a more tangible form.

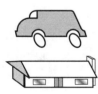

Let's determine the number of small $10,000 cars that that would buy? The answer is, 100 million.

It represents ten million $100,000 homes.

That is also equivalent to one million people each winning a one million dollar prize at the lottery.

Or to put it still another way, with the money spent on healthcare in the United States, we could feed every American for an entire year.

Make up your own example!

Ten	10^1
10	
Hundred	10^2
100	
10x10	
Thousand	10^3
1,000	
10x10x10	
Million	10^6
1,000,000	
1,000 x thousand	
1,000 x 1,000	
Billion	10^9
1,000,000,000	
1,000 x million	
1,000 x 1,000 x 1,000	
Trillion	10^{12}
1,000,000,000,000	
1,000 x billion	
1,000 x 1,000 x 1,000 x 1,000	

At the family level

This individual figure of $3,000 applies to each and every person in the United States, including children, parents and the elderly. Therefore, for a family with two children it costs $12,000 a year for their health insurance. That is want it costs. Whether it be paid through an employer, direct contributions, or income taxes, it is still we who pay it in its entirety.

If we wished, we could pay a doctor $100,000 a year to look after the health needs of 32 individuals or of eight families of four on a full time basis. Just imagine the personalized service we could get.

There would be a lot less sickness around! The doctor would soon realize that it would be in his or her best interest to ensure that we are healthy if for no other reason than to have as much time as possible to follow a leisure pursuit, like playing golf, for example. The doctor would discover very quickly the benefits of the medicine of health. Why shouldn't we treat ourselves to this luxury, considering all the money we are spending?

At the personal level

As few of us actually pay these costs directly, these figures may seem afford-able at first glance. Remember, however, that it is the minority of the population that absorbs these costs. The rich, the elderly, children and those who are out of work do not contribute. For those who are working, it is a question of them paying much more than just for their families. Clever calculations have been done which show that **we work approximately three-and-a-half months** (3 ½) a year solely to pay for our health insurance! Think about it. Three-and-a-half months for the privilege of being sick. No wonder that we are.

WHERE DOES OUR MONEY GO?

What is it that costs so much? We only have to look at what we spend the most on when we go to see a doctor.

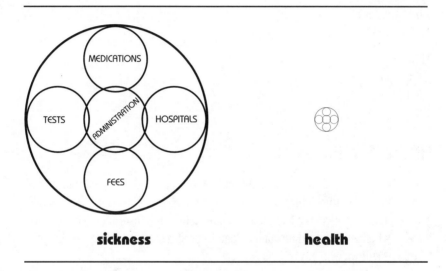

sickness   **health**

1) Diagnostic tests

Laboratory tests, X-rays, early detection, scanning, biopsies and all the new tests that are more and more sophisticated. These tests are used for everything and nothing. They are often repeated. They require extremely expensive equip-ment and specialized operators who are also expensive. The equipment always has to be the latest model, rather like cars. It is now ingrained in the mentality of doctors that they cannot diagnose a patient without equipment, and the latest at that, and without resorting to one or more tests.

Doctors often order these tests before even examining their patient. It is customary, for example, for a cardiologist to automatically conduct an electro-cardiogram the moment the patient enters the office. Whether it is necessary or not. A hospital will be judged based on the **quantity** of state-of-the-art techno-logical equipment it has. And not on the **quality** of its services to patients.

TESTS COST AN ARM AND A LEG

2) Medicines and drugs

While we may not always leave our doctor's office with a form for a test, we hardly ever leave without a prescription in hand. It has come to the point where, if our doctor fails to write such a prescription, then we wouldn't consider him to be a very good doctor. We would lose confidence in him. And we would go and see another.

When complications and after-effects occur, we go right back to the doctor who prescribes another medication to counter the bad effects of the first. And we take twice as much. And then three times as much, and so on, up to 20 pills at a time for many elderly people. They are so drugged that many fall and fracture their hip!

MEDICATIONS COST AN ARM AND A LEG

3) Hospitals

You don't have to try and figure out what is most expensive in hospitals. Everything is! They represent about 50% of the entire health insurance costs. Hospital clients, to a large degree, are there for sophisticated tests. Above all, remember that one hospitalization in three is caused by after effects of medication. It therefore becomes obvious that hospital costs are directly proportional to our use of diagnostic tests and medications.

HOSPITALS COST AND ARM AND A LEG

4) Other costs

One can also guess that these include the professional fees that relate directly to the services we receive and the administrative costs, which are directly proportional to the overall medical costs.

CONCLUSION

So-called health systems are systems of sickness.

Doctors are only concerned with sickness.

Yet, **sickness costs an arm and a leg!**

Then, we must find a solution. And fast.

The solution:
a medicine of health

WHAT IS HEALTH?

According to the conventions of scientific medicine, health is "the absence of sickness". To be healthy, means that **one is not sick**. This very practical definition applies in many cases. However, how does one explain a heart attack suffered by someone whose tests proved normal? Take a woman who has felt out of sorts, experiencing some minor discomfort. She goes to see her doctor. She is put through a battery of physical and laboratory tests. Only to be told: "Don't worry. Everything is normal."

How can she suddenly die, "in good health", the very next week? How can one explain such a thing? To be in perfect health one day and dead the next? Unless, of course, one has a serious accident. Can one pass from being healthy to being dead, from one day to the next? Yes, if one refers to the conventional definition of health. No, if one defines health in another manner: variable health or the "health-thermometer."

Health-thermometer

Since **health is a continuum** along which our state of health varies, we should be able to measure it using an imaginary thermometer ranging from 0 to 100 percent. The higher the better. When high, one is said to be healthy, the light zone. Less, and one is said to be less healthy, the grey zone. When not healthy at all, one enters the black zone.

One day, we might be at 50 percent, the next at 52. Our health can also vary several degrees when we experience a big emotional shock. For example, one can suddenly drop from 65 to 40, and can continue to deteriorate to the point where an illness manifests itself. The patient who "died in good health", as mentioned earlier, was not healthy at all. She had probably entered the black zone on the scale without any measurable signs of illness. But she was ill. And she was gravely ill at that.

How many times have we heard people say after they had gone to see their doctor because they were not feeling well or felt ill: "My doctor told me that there was nothing wrong with me. I was in perfect shape. That I had nothing to

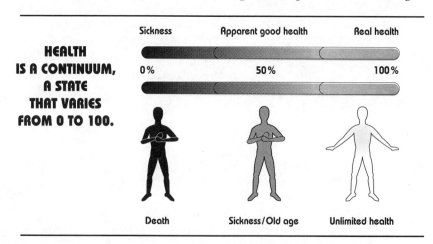

HEALTH IS A CONTINUUM, A STATE THAT VARIES FROM 0 TO 100.

Sickness	Apparent good health	Real health
0%	50%	100%

| Death | Sickness/Old age | Unlimited health |

worry about". Had the doctor lied? No. He gave an evaluation conforming to the scientific definition of health. However, I believe a definition along the scale of a "health-thermometer" to be more appropriate. It better translates reality.

How then can we evaluate health? How can we know our exact position on the scale between 0 and 100? While nothing has ever really been established in this regard, I would like to make the following analogy.

Let's take the example of a used car. Are we going to check the principal systems and, if there is no evident problem (no illness), conclude that the car is in excellent shape (perfect health), and pay 100% of its value? No. We take it for a test drive, listen to the engine, and then check out that the brakes work (physical exam).

We ask about the history and maintenance of the car over the past few years. Who had driven it? Where? How? With tender loving care? Or as a hot rod with total abandon? Was the oil changed regularly with a good quality product? Was the body washed and polished on a regular basis? Did it receive an anti-rust treatment? Was it ever driven over dirt roads? Was it subjected to a lot of stop and go traffic? Was it involved in an accident? Only when one adds up the answers to all these questions, can one determine whether the car is in good or bad shape. And only then is the price determined accordingly.

The same goes for health. Apart from physical and laboratory tests, one must evaluate the other aspects of the person's lifestyle. The person who eats fast-food, sleeps four hours a night, smokes three packets of cigarettes a day, works under stress 12 hours a day, and who regularly downs five scotches and a bottle of wine, is potentially not in good health. But surprising as it might seem, the same person could be in better health than the "health nut" stuck in a job he doesn't like simply because the job provides him with security.

Then there is the person who doesn't drink much, who takes care of herself, but works in a job that places tremendous pressure on her. She too is not in good health. And soon she will be suffering from heartburn, migraine headaches, and back pains. Or she happens to be someone who is always trying to please others to the detriment of her innermost self, she is not in good health either. Tomorrow, she will be told she has a cancer, but she will never understand why it came about.

The other advantage of defining health along the scale of a "health-thermometer" is that it permits a continual improvement. People will assume that if they are not sick: "I'm in good health, therefore I can act just as I want, accept any pressure along the way, and do whatever I wish." Right up until the day they suddenly crack up, again without ever knowing why. If we use our "health-thermometer" as a definition, we will come to better understand our state of health. We can prevent the catastrophe and, above all, continuously improve our state of health.

Inevitable death

In the **materialistic** optic in which we live, life begins with birth, and ends with death. We achieve the maximum "degrees" of health at about the age of 20 and

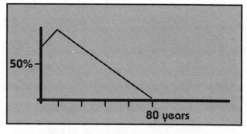

then our body begins to tire, wear out, and we are on an inevitable downhill slope to sickness, aging, and death.

Sickness, suffering, aging and death are the consequences of thought limited in time and space. Everything is built around this. Health insurance, life (death) insurance, retirement, pension funds, prepaid funeral services, etc. We are robots programmed to be born and then to obey, study, work, consume, become old, and die. The path is already mapped out for us and we follow it. We submit ourselves to our fate. We endure our lot in life and we do so without complaining. Awaiting our final deliverance.

We are a throw-away disposable commodity, just like any other on this planet.

Unlimited health

From a spiritualistic perspective, on the other hand, our earthly life is but a step in our eternal life. Our spirit has always been and always will be. Forever. It is perfect health.

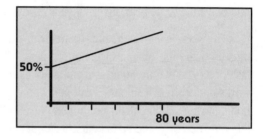

In quantum physics, time and space are illusions. They do not exist. Their corollaries, sickness, aging and death are also illusions and not realities. They can only exist if we believe them to exist. So we give them body in tangible form.

The state of health of our physical body is going to depend upon to what degree it is in harmony with the spirit. If the body is one with the spirit, it will vibrate at the same frequency and it will come to know the perfect and eternal health that the spirit now enjoys.

Health improves continually, from one day to the next and from one incarnation to another incarnation. Even death is a step of growth.

This choice between the two points of view stems from our inner power to choose, which is to be found in the soul. It is the centre of conscience and the will. It is sovereign. It regulates and frees the emission of energy flow in our body, following its own state of health. The soul is sovereign of the body.

N.B. For reasons of simplicity, I will use the words Health to mean good health and Sickness to mean poor health.

WHAT IS SICKNESS?

Sickness occurs when the body shows its disharmony with the soul. They are no longer on the same wavelength. And this disharmony is blocking the transmission of the vibrations of our spirit and is preventing them from spreading throughout our entire body. Sickness is a physical manifestation of a much deeper problem. Sickness is always seen as a misfortune that happens, out of the blue, by chance, attributable to an exterior agent.

Congratulations

Whenever my friends fall ill, I send them a card which reads: "Congratulations on your illness and don't get well too soon."

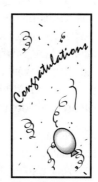

Because I believe that sickness is an information, and an opportunity we give ourselves.

Let me explain. Illness is the language our body uses to tell us that it is upset, physically and morally. As a matter of fact, more and more, people are taking note of the importance of the inter-relationship between morale (emotions/thoughts) and the physical bodies. We know that the sickness of one can induce a sickness in the other. For example, a great sadness (morale) can lead to a cancer (physical).

It is the same for the cause and the treatment. Taking care of one improves the other. And vice versa. Someone who is paralyzed and begins to walk again has his morale lifted with each step. It is at the very root of psychosomatic medicine (psycho = psyche; Somos = Greek for body), and of the "holistic" approach to medicine (global medicine).

Sickness, in such a context, is the manifestation of a physical, emotional, mental, or spiritual problem. It provides us with information. It sets off an alarm bell. How lucky we are to have it! Providing, of course, that we listen to it and we know how to use it. Our reaction, in the face of illness, can be one of two kinds:

- either we see it as an enemy, we curse it, and we shut it off with surgery or drugs. We simply negate it. But it will come back knocking at our door. Sooner or later.

- or we look upon it as an ally. We rush to decode the message which it has transmitted to us. And we try to resolve the real cause of the problem.

Again, let us look at the car. As soon as we hear a strange noise, we rush to the garage and ask them to check it out. They will look for the cause in order to fix the real problem before the car breaks down and we are stuck somewhere. "Take the time that you need to figure out the real cause of the problem so that it is fixed and will not create another problem elsewhere."

When it comes to ourselves, we rush to take an aspirin for a headache. An anti-acid tablet for heartburn. Or a *Valium* for nerves. All to get as far away from the pain as possible. It will come back and we start taking the pills again. Until finally, the "breakdown" occurs. That is to say the illness which forces us to stop our activities. Will we again rush off to be operated on or submit to treatment without asking ourselves what is the real origin of this illness? For the information is there. If we do not, we are going to have all the time in the world to think about it during our convalescence. But think about what?

Thinking about what?

In our society, it is still considered better to go and see a doctor than a psychologist.

Think of the real reasons why we are so deeply disturbed and which have forced us to come to a halt. We don't like our job any more. Our relationship with our partner is dead. Our children or our friends treat us badly. Our father or mother terrorizes us. We are fed up with having to work for a living. The competition is killing us. And so on, and so on. We refuse to think about it. For if we did, then we would have to do something to remedy the situation. And that makes us afraid. Afraid of what? Fear of changing one's job, fear of divorce, that our children will love us less or tell others that we are bad parents, fear of guilt, etc.

Sickness is the equivalent of divorce, a heartbreak, being stuck in a rut professionally, or bankruptcy. It is precipitated by the loss of respect from someone who is dear to us, the loss of a job, the loss of money, the death of a loved one, a move, etc. All these situations have a common denominator. We fear change. Change that we push aside and avoid until it really makes us sick. We would rather stay in bed than face up to the real situation. We blame the heavens, fate, our boss, and just about everyone else in the world, except for ourselves. We consult a doctor, we make the pain go away, and the real reason that caused us to fall ill in the first place is not addressed.

"People die at 25 years old, but they are not buried until they are 75!"

Security is death.

If only we could maintain the status quo! We are prepared to remain half well, or half ill, rather than face the real underlying problems because they disturb us. They threaten our security.

And let's talk about security! What is this term which causes us to accept so much suffering? An illusion!

Let us look at one example that we are always hearing about and one that saddens me. Security in the workplace, or job security. I know a number of teachers, for example, who no longer want to teach because they were never really cut out for the job in the first place, or because they would welcome a change and the chance to practice another profession? But they remain prisoners of their wage security. They have been made to believe that their employer, the State, will never go bankrupt.

All they have to do is "hang in" in order to have a guaranteed salary, with cost of living increases, and retirement benefits at the end of the line. Isn't that just great? And so, while they are hanging in there, they put up with headaches, back aches, depression, and digestive problems. Their body is crying out that it can't take it any more, that it doesn't like this way of life, that it wants to do something else.

But they "keep hanging in there". There is no way they are going to give up their job security. Better to be sick than to be insecure about one's job. One day, they will become so ill that they will have to stop working. But they held up well. They made it long enough to take an early retirement, before dying, surrounded by all that security. They were dead the day they gave up their soul for job security.

Realigning one's sights

Sickness is a malfunction of the soul. If we wish to profit from it, we have to see it as an ally that we have called upon to help us realign our sights, and refind our direction. That is to say that:

1. We are responsible for our sickness and we caused it to come about, albeit unconsciously. We are therefore masters of the situation. And not victims of events or other people.

2. We got lost along the way and we want to regain our direction - our goal in life - why we are on Earth. It is the spiritual aspect of health which is unfortunately so rarely considered. And yet, it is so paramount.

Taking a trip, going for a ride in a car, is all very well. But one must know where one wants to go, if one is to choose the right direction to take. Such is the purpose of sickness. To remind us of exactly that.

> **"Don't climb the ladder of success only to find it's leaning against the wrong wall."**
> Bernie Siegel

WHAT IS A DOCTOR?

Doctors are human beings. They eat three times a day. They sleep. They worry, celebrate, get irritable, laugh, cry, love, hate. They argue with their loved ones, get angry with their children, worry about their finances. They have their fears and insecurities. In brief, they survive.

A doctor is a product of our society, with an image created to conform to that society. As in any field or profession, there are good, average, and mediocre ones. Neither saints nor sinners, still less gods, all are human.

In general, when doctors start on their careers, they are full of good intentions with noble ideals. The majority have chosen this profession to help others. Some to acquire respectability and/or to please their parents. Others, finally, to ensure financial comfort. There are, of course, those who do it for a combination of reasons.

Doctors are no different from their patients. Except for one little detail. We have spent from four to ten years, sometimes more, in a medical school and a hospital where it was ingrained in us that:

- The role of the doctor is to heal and save lives.
- Sickness and death represent defeats. The doctor must avoid them at all cost.
- The medical education and training received is the only valid one. The doctor is in possession of the truth.

- Doctors always have an answer for any question and must know everything. If there is something they don't know, it is because it does not exist.

- Doctors are workhorses, working 15 hours a day. That's normal, they are, after all, superhuman.

- Statistics are infallible, or almost. They must be believed and followed, if one is to remain scientific and thorough.

- Patients act like statistics and must follow the recommendations of the doctor in full confidence, blindly.

- Doctors cannot get involved emotionally. They must remain cold and aloof in order to keep control of the situation and make logical decisions.

- The doctor is the god of health. All other practitioners are inferior.

- Doctors are part of the elite of society.

Getting Doctored
Martin Shapiro

And we believed it! Some still do. Others have their doubts. Others no longer believe it at all. I am one of the latter. I entered medicine full of ideals. I knew the golden era of medicine, if I may put it that way. That is to say, the time when we had succeeded, one believed, in controlling the principal illnesses. Illnesses such as tuberculosis, diphtheria, infections. One no longer died of appendicitis. We now operated on the heart. We seemed unbeatable and invincible. There were still some cancers or stubborn, hard-to-beat arthritis, but it was only a question of time before we would have them too under control. We had not yet even heard of AIDS.

In light of such successes, and such a rosy picture, how could we not enthusiastically adopt the teaching we received? Yes, I believed it. I believed it for many years. Before realizing that I did not have all the answers. Neither did the learned books or leading experts. I had to learn to say, in all honesty: "I do not know" and, to my amazement, my patients didn't hold it against me. On the contrary.

I also detected that emotional and mental problems exerted a strong influence on the health of my patients. That concern or worry caused headaches or heartburn. That I could accept. But when my patient suffered from pain in the legs (I am a phlebologist) without any physical problem to explain it, other than she was going through a divorce, well that was powerful stuff!

From illusion to reality

I therefore began to doubt the sanctity of medical truth. My faith was shaken. I began asking myself questions and visiting doctors, non-doctors, healers, researchers in several countries, as far away as Siberia. I noticed the extraordinary results they were achieving through their methods.

I came into contact with the parallel world of health. One on which the all-powerful establishment was stomping despite the fact that they were doing their patients good. I realized that there was a very strong hierarchy in medicine. And I understood why, very early on, they had put us doctors on a pedestal and taught us to mistrust all non-doctors. Why they treated therapists as charlatans, chiropractors as exploiters, psychologists as unbalanced, and nurses as 'Jills-of-all-trade'.

Today, I no longer believe the sanctity of medical truth. Yet, in a way, I believe more than ever. I believe in a wealth of knowledge which is to be found beyond that which we were taught. The conscience. I believe in the all-powerful nature of the medicine which is to be found within each of us. I believe in well-informed and responsible patients who will know how to take charge of their health and govern it accordingly. With our support and encouragement. I believe in doctors and therapists who work together in close collaboration, and who will rediscover the enthusiasm they once had. As well as love for their profession.

AT MEDICAL SCHOOL, I LEARNED
WITH MY PATIENTS, I UNDERSTOOD

WHAT IS MEDICINE?

Medicine is:

- a science, the objective of which is preserving and restoring health.
- the art of preventing and caring for human illnesses. But above all, THE ART OF LIVING

A science and an art

When one speaks of vibrations or biochemical reactions, one speaks of science. Science, notably physics, has its laws which are totally applicable to biology. However, the human being is also made up of subtle components that one cannot see or touch. It is the artist, and their perceptive talents, that we call upon to interpret these bodies in visual form.

Medicine is therefore a science and an art, all at the same time. It calls upon our sensorial and rational knowledge, as well as upon our extra-sensorial and intuitive perception.

In other times, before the advent of our patriarchal society, medicine was often practiced by midwives. In French, they are called *"sage-femmes"*, the word *sage* meaning wise. They were so called because they were recognized for their wisdom in their community. They had established a tradition of healing based on wisdom. But they were treated as witches and were burned.

> **Healing Wise**
> Susun S. Weed

This tradition, the *Wise Woman Tradition*, is marvelously well explained and given respectability once again, by Susun Weed in her book: ***Healing Wise.*** I love the first words of the Wise Woman when faced with a health problem. Namely,*"do nothing"*. It reminds me of a Latin phrase that I have heard, *"Primum non nocere"* which means, in essence, "Above all, do not be prejudicial". I am afraid that we have forgotten.

Three bodies, three medicines

As the spirit is the Light, it is always in good health. It doesn't need medicine. It is THE medicine. It is the principle of all healing. That is why:

- healing rests entirely with those who are experiencing the suffering.

All other medicine is only a complementary aid to help patients work on themselves.

So that we are all clear on the terms, I will try here, far from perfectly I might add, to distinguish the three main therapeutic approaches which are available to us. And I will also add the essential characteristics of each. I have categorized them according to their main field. But remember that these often overlap one another. It is the same with practitioners. Medicine is not the sole purview of any one person or group, be they doctors, therapists, or healers.

Isn't the only real doctor the patient?

MEDICINE	SCIENTIFIC	ALTERNATIVE	SELF-HEALING	
PRINCIPAL TARGET:	visible body	invisible body	soul	spirit
SEAT OF:	physical	emotions thoughts	conscience	
SYSTEM:	death	survival	life	
PART OF PROBLEM APPROACHED:	manifestation of problem	problem itself	cause of problem	
DEFINITION:	science	art	faith in oneself	
FIELD OF ACTION:	reductionist (symptomatic)	holistic	unlimited	never
OBJECTIVE:	kill the sickness	maintain health	improve health	
ACTION:	war (attack)	defense	peace	
MEANS:	medications and surgery which destroy	remedies which clean and reinforce	unconditional love which nourishes	sick
EFFECTS:	treats the sickness	takes care of the one who is sick	empowers the person	treats
DURATION OF EFFECT:	temporary	lasting	permanent	
COSTS:	$$$$$	$¢	❤	health
PRACTITIONER:	doctor	therapist	oneself	
ATTITUDE TOWARDS THE SICKNESS:	enemy	punishment	ally	unlimited
ATTITUDE OF PRACTITIONER TOWARDS THE PATIENT:	a number	human being	co-creator	
ATTITUDE OF PATIENT TOWARDS PRACTITIONER:	obeys authority	questions authority	is the authority	
INVOLVEMENT OF PATIENT:	dependence	participation	sovereignty	
PREVENTION:	detect and treat early on	maintain and improve health	raise level of health	
RESULT	aggravation	improvement	cure	

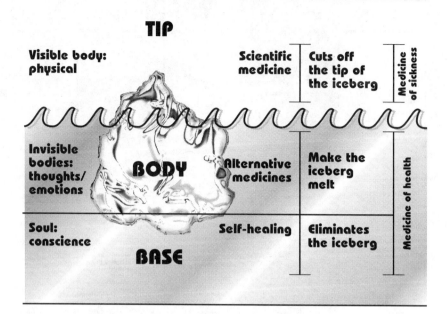

Scientific medicine for the physical body

It is the medicine that we all know. It is practiced by doctors trained in university medical schools. Scientific medicine is based on the materialistic physics of Newton. Such a cause gives such an effect. A given symptom coming from a given illness requires a given treatment. The anticipated results conform with the given statistics.

It recognizes only that which it can see, touch, and measure. The truth is only to be found in tests. **Science** makes the law. It therefore automatically denies the existence of invisible bodies. And the same is true of all links between the emotions, thought, conscience, and state of health of the physical body. Whenever it is confronted with a problem of this kind, it slaps on a "psychosomatic" label and patients are sent home with pills for their nerves.

For scientific medicine, which is essentially materialistic, life begins with birth and ends with death. One must avoid the latter at all cost. The death of a patient is a defeat for the doctor.

Also according to scientific medicine, illness is always an aggressive agent coming from the exterior. A microbe, tumor, pain, etc. They must be fought and war is declared. War on cancer, battling AIDS, wiping out epidemics (vaccines), eliminating pain with pain-killers. Quite a military vocabulary, wouldn't you say, and an arsenal of attack. It is the medicine of war. And like war, scientific medicine is **destructive, extremely costly,** and **doesn't solve anything.**

Destructive

According to Harris Coulter, "authorities have estimated that adverse reactions related to prescribed medicines cause or contribute to one-third of all deaths in the United States every year (700,000 out of 2 million deaths annually)." Add to that deaths and secondary effects related to surgery and other aggressive treatments such as radiotherapy. Without forgetting debilitating treatments such as those practiced in psychiatric hospitals where patients are quite literally imprisoned. This medical bludgeoning disconnects them from their soul and prevents them from living their sickness. Therefore, they can never be healed. And they remain forever prisoners, dependent upon drugs and medication.

Medicines and drugs are legalized poisons

You have probably already asked yourself why **synthetic medicines** *cause adverse, negative reactions, while* **natural remedies** *(physiotherapy, homeopathy) have no secondary effects? The answer is simple.*

- *Medicines and drugs are synthetic products that cannot be assimilated by the organism (we can't digest plastic, for example). They* **work against nature**. *Be that as it may, the authorities impose scientific medicine which places priority on the use of medicines and drugs. They spread* **(dis)order**.

- *Remedies are natural products that can be assimilated by the organism (one can digest plants, for example). They* **work with nature**. *And yet, the authorities prohibit alternative medicines which use these remedies. They refuse* **order**.

Extremely costly

As is the case with war, scientific medicine requires very sophisticated and costly equipment. Yet in all reality, it is very rare that one really needs very elaborate tests. Some 95% of tests could be avoided, either because they are unnecessary, or because they could be postponed to a later date. The evolution of the sick person almost always provides the answer. Even a so-called emergency may not be one if it doesn't require immediate intervention.

The diagnostic skill rests with the patients, not with machines. Let us question and examine them. And then question again and re-examine. They will give us the answer on a silver platter. What the patients need, is to be reassured that they are not about to die. It doesn't call for an immediate diagnostic test. But scientific medicine imposes it upon the patient. And the patient believes that the best hospital is the one with the best machines.

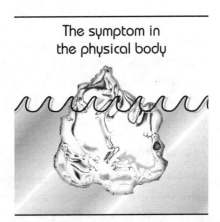

The symptom in the physical body

It solves nothing

Scientific medicine makes the symptom or the sign of the body disappear. It doesn't cure it. It only shears off the tip of the iceberg. But the problem, the bulk of the iceberg, remains. And the tip will grow again, sooner or later.

Let us take, for example, a headache. It is the symptom which leads a patient to consult a doctor. If the patient is given something to relieve it, then the headache will go away. Only to return once the effect has worn off. As the cause of the headache remains, it will come back even stronger and more frequently. The same thing for surgery. Removing an organ does not correct the cause.

As it does not cure the cause, scientific medicine keeps the patient in a state of dependence and permanent submission.

Beware of the octopus!

Scientific medicine is an octopus that we are not afraid of, or distrust, because we only see a little part at a time. The tip of a tentacle. We forget that being caught by the tentacle can mean the beginning of the end. It always tries to draw its victim near in order to devour it.

*A patient told me one day that she was going to have an operation on her elbow. I asked her if surgery was really necessary and whether she had considered other alternative solutions. She told me yes. She had consulted three people. And all three had recommended surgery. I then asked her who these three people were. "The three best orthopedists in the city," she replied. I mentioned to her that a surgeon recommends what he knows best. Surgery! He could not recommend something he knew nothing about. The patient then realized that a "**second opinion**" in scientific medicine is simply a repeat of the first opinion.*

When we go to a doctor for whatever reason whatsoever, we may not realize that we are coming within the reach of the tentacles, the arms of the medical system. From one ordinary test for an ordinary problem, it will find something which seems to be ordinary. It will then do another test, more complicated this time, to ensure that it is really an ordinary problem, and when it again gives an ordinary result, "We're not sure. We will have to take more tests." Now we really begin to worry. As the tests increase, so does our fear. The octopus has us in its grasp. We want out? We want to stop everything and escape? Yes, **but...** that **but** has already condemned us.

In conclusion

Scientific medicine should only be used in the last resort, when all else has failed. And that is true of both the diagnostic equipment and treatment. Except for emergencies, which goes without saying. It is not that doctors are rotten or corrupt. The fault lies with the medical system they serve.

Good family doctors, full of common sense and compassion, have kept their sense of proper judgement. They don't follow the doctrine set down by the authorities and don't allow themselves to be influenced by the threat of possible legal action. They listen to their patients and propose simple and effective solutions. They help their patients to feel better about themselves and to do what needs to be done.

This type of doctor does exist. We all know one. They don't need a title or a degree. Everyone respects them for their wisdom. It is by listening to our heart, our feelings, that we will make the choice between doctors who practice dogmatic scientific medicine and those who practice a medicine of common sense and compassion.

Alternative medicines for the invisible bodies

These are the medicines which we are hearing more and more of nowadays. They are also called energetic medicines, vibratory medicines, natural therapies, parallel medicines, alternative medicines, complementary medicines, and holistic medicines. In general, they are taught in non-university specialized schools. They are based on quantum physics and recognize the existence of invisible bodies.

Alternative therapies are practiced by therapists who are knowledgeable of energy and vibrations. The most often practiced therapies are chiropractic, kinesiology, osteopathy, homeopathy, acupuncture, and naturopathy. To these we can add psychotherapy, massotherapy, and phytotherapy. Healers are in a category all of their own. They work directly on energy. They are gifted with very special talents.

Contrary to scientific medicine which takes care of the illness, alternative medicines take care of **the one who is sick**. They focus on reinforcing one's natural defenses. They work to improve the overall state of health of patients so that they themselves, in their turn, can defend themselves against any harmful agent.

Alternative medicines work at two levels:

a) on the invisible bodies. The sickness attains the invisible bodies before it manifests itself in the visible physical body. It therefore makes sense to first of all treat the invisible bodies, the hidden part of the iceberg.

b) on the visible physical body in order to help it while waiting for improvement brought about by the treatment of the invisible bodies.

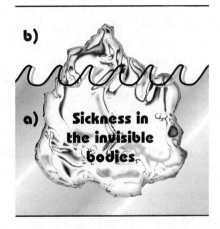

b)

a) Sickness in the invisible bodies.

In general, alternative medicines do not cause side effects. The best example of this is homeopathy, which some now call the medicine of the 21st Century. I have seen marvelous results in very many cases, particularly relating to allergies and otitis in children. All of the chronic problems. It even improves one's character.

Alternative medicines are custom-made for each patient because the cause of the problem differs from one patient to the next, even if the symptoms are the same. From time to time, they require the input of a therapist. They are much less expensive than scientific medicine. In addition, they regulate the problem in depth. They free patients and encourage them to become autonomous.

Holistic medicine

These consider the human being as a whole, made up of a body, a soul, and a spirit. At the same time, they use words in a sense that is different to what we have seen above:

The body   =   the physical body
                 (visible: treated primarily by osteopathy)

The soul   =   the body of emotions
                 (invisible: treated primarily by homeopathy)

The spirit =   the body of thoughts
                 (invisible: treated primarily by acupuncture)

As the bodies are inter-dependent, any treatment of one leads to improvement of the others. Re-establishing the health of an affected organ also corrects the imbalance that has been triggered in the organism.

Complementary medicine

This combines scientific medicine and alternative medicines. It is practiced by doctors who have added one or more alternative medicine practices to their existing scientific medicine arsenal. At first glance, that may seem like getting the best of two worlds. But it is rarely the case. "Clothes do not make the man", as the old saying goes.

The two practices, scientific medicine and alternative medicines, are diametrically opposed. One cannot mix fire and water. The two elements are all-important in their own right, but they can never be mixed together. A doctor may be interested in alternative medicines but, if he practices them, he will do so in a scientific manner. He will treat the symptoms rather than reinforcing the overall state of the patient. A doctor who is really "converted" to alternative medicines will never be able to practice scientific medicine again. It will no longer make sense. Unfortunately, doctors often adopt alternative medicines for purely financial reasons instead of referring patients to those whose field it is.

TRUE complementary medicine does exist. It is that which brings together around a table, the patient, therapist, and doctor. It is the patient who leads the discussion. The patient takes the decision - enlightened - and decides what steps to follow for the treatment, or non-treatment. It is a partnership for the benefit of the patient.

These small, multi-disciplinary collaborative groups are growing in number. Always bear in mind that the only "doctor is the patient."

Self-healing for the soul

One hardly ever hears of this medicine, also known as spiritual medicine. It is easy to understand why.

- First of all, because the soul is poorly understood, or not at all. Scientific doctors deny its existence. Therapists know it exists, but don't know what to do with it. The soul is an enigma. And yet...

- Secondly, because according to tradition, religion took care of the soul. A lay person would undoubtedly have been burned alive at the stake if he or she had committed such a sacrilege. But times have changed. We are now free of religious powers and it is spiritual masters who teach us spirituality and the health of the soul. We have to be careful, however, not to replace our former religious leaders with masters or gurus. That will not be any better. Whether you obey one doctrine or another, the result is the same. Submission to an external power.

- Thirdly, because there is a very big step to make in order to pass from alternative medicines to self-healing. As big as passing from scientific medicine to alternative medicines. This step requires a new transformation of consciousness with all the difficulties that this entails.

Medicine of the soul is practiced individually or in a group. New techniques are being developed which address the soul directly. They are very efficient. The results are there... for those who really want to change their level of consciousness.

Sicknesses of the conscience: a lack of memory

These are the most frequent sicknesses which prevent the conscience from growing and changing.

1. **Victimization**
   Victims are put upon, dominated, exploited. They can do nothing about it and are not responsible for anything. They can only blame external factors such as circumstances, people, etc. We **forget** that we are sovereign.

2. **Securization**
   Those who are well off are particularly prone. They are afraid of losing their job, money, love, etc. They will make themselves ill rather than give up their illusion of security. Job security is a malignant form. We **forget** that we are rich, even if we don't own anything.

3. Protectionism

Another illness which causes us to give up our sovereignty to external powers to compensate for the low opinion that we have of ourselves. We **forget** that we are all-powerful.

4. Normopathy

The sickness of those who always follow the norm. Who think like everyone else. Who say what everyone else is saying. Who act like everyone else. Mr. Everyone, the man in the street, is sick. He is suffering from normopathy. It is a contagious sickness which is passed on to those around him, from family to family, from region to region. It is to live through proxy, rather than living what one really is with all that this entails in terms of differences and originality. It is to become a carbon copy of others, living an illusion. We **forget** that we are unique and divine.

In each case, our conscience is paralyzed by fear or imprisoned in belief. We have **forgotten** our inner divinity.

No self-health without self-sickness

From spectators to actors

Going from being a spectator to becoming an actor is a transformation. It consists of quitting our role of being a spectator of our life. We must stop being passive in front of events that arrive and putting them down to fate. We recognize that we are responsible actors for all that happens to us. We take our life in hand and master our own destiny, living it how we wish to live it. We create our future. We become the authors of our life.

Victimization and all its faults give way to responsibility. We can write it in such a way that it is a great story. With a happy ending!

Patients take control of their health. They know that they alone can heal themselves and have faith in their divinity. They also know that nobody else can do this for them. Doctors and therapists can only help make them aware, accompany them. They also know that sickness is an opportunity to readjust and give a new direction to their life. They take advantage of it by making it their ally.

"The real doctor is the doctor within. Most doctors know nothing of this science and yet it works so well."

Albert Schweitzer

In conclusion

Self-healing is the process of transformation of the conscience. It works on the base of the iceberg and melts it progressively and surely until it disappears entirely. It is the only medicine that CURES, that is to say which cures the root of the problem once and for all.

IT IS IN THE SOUL
THAT SICKNESS IS BORN...
SO TOO IS THE CURE!

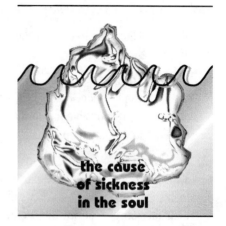

the cause
of sickness
in the soul

A MEDICINE OF HEALTH

Medicine of health re-establishes, maintains and increases health. It takes care, on one hand, of the invisible bodies which is a medicine of improvement, and on the other, the medicine of self-healing. In every instance, it raises the level of consciousness.

Practicing a medicine of improvement is to put emphasis on the factors which **maintain** and **re-establish** health.	Practicing a medicine of self-healing is to put emphasis on the factors which **increase** health.
It is a medicine which:	It is a medicine which:
• gives priority to health over sickness.	• definitely cures.
• recognizes the existence of the soul and the body.	• recognizes the priority of the soul over the body.
• corrects the problem rather than the symptoms.	• corrects the cause of the problem.
• encourages the patient to become autonomous.	• encourages the patient to become sovereign.
• discourages consumerism.	• does not involve consumerism.
It is the medicine of invisible bodies.	It is the medicine of the soul. It transforms the consciousness.

One day, I received a call from a woman living some distance away explaining that she had just opened a health center and that she was looking for a doctor to work there. So I asked her whether it was a center of sickness that she had opened. No, health, she replied, obviously astonished at my question. I then asked her why she wanted to hire a doctor, given the fact that doctors only treat illnesses, not health. Realizing the difference, she stopped looking.

The invisible exists

The medicine of health recognizes that the invisible exists. We are more than just robots in flesh and blood. Our thoughts and emotions greatly influence our state of health, even if they cannot be seen. Our consciousness gives us the power to direct and live our life as we wish. That it is freedom of choice which distinguishes us from the animals.

Moreover, animals also have emotions that can affect their state of health, as well as plants, as has been clearly demonstrated by Christopher Bird and Peter Tomkins in their book: **The Secret Life of Plants.**

We instinctively know just how much our emotions and our thoughts influence our daily health and how they can harm it.

It wasn't by accident that Bernie Siegel's book: **Love, Medicine and Miracles** was such a phenomenal success. In addition to having been written by a man of great compassion, this book brings to the fore that which we know in our innermost selves. It confirms our daily experiences and explains to us why sicknesses respond differently to identical treatments. It confirms that we are not machines and that, above all, we need love. It is all very well to talk about love. But one cannot buy it, or see it. It is invisible. And yet, it is essential to life!

Another doctor who has also touched on the problem, but from an angle that is more scientific than practical, is Deepak Chopra. In his best-seller: **Quantum Healing - Exploring the Frontiers of Mind/Body Medicine,** he provides us with the explanation that we are looking for. He follows through on his study of quantum physics to conclude that eternal youth is possible. He goes on sharing his secrets with us in his most recent book: **Timeless Mind, Ageless Body**.

A scientist, Beverly Rubik has also written a most interesting book on the frontiers of the visible and the invisible entitled: **The Interrelationship Between Mind and Matter.**

> **Love, Medicine and Miracles**
> Bernie Siegel

There are many others in the world to show that the invisible exists and that sickness appears in the invisible bodies before manifesting itself in the physical body. Yet in spite of everything, scientific medicine continues to deny it. Up until the time we were plunged into "scientific" materialism, which reduces us to physico-chemical reactions, the invisible was recognized and was revered and treated with respect. Once people were ostracized, who did not have faith in the invisible. Nowadays, one terrorizes those who do.

Identifying the problem: the invisible bodies

A symptom is only the tip of the iceberg. It is the small external manifestation of a deeper and bigger problem that we cannot see well below the surface.

WHAT IS THE REAL PROBLEM?

The story of a commonplace occurrence that follows illustrates well how our organism functions and how each organ compensates for the lack of the other in providing additional help in order to maintain overall balance. **When the physical sickness appears**, it is because the real problem has been dragging on for some time without ever having been resolved. And that the entire organism is exhausted. The symptom cannot reveal the real problem. We must dig deep to find the problem itself. Often, the symptom is deceptive and misleading. The problem turns out to be much different to that which the symptom appears to indicate. The symptom only serves to warn us: "Look deeper. There is a problem below!"

When we seek, we invariably discover just how much false thoughts and beliefs imprison us. And how fear paralyzes us. Beliefs and fear rule in a materialistic world. They impose their heavy vibes on the more vulnerable physical body. It suffers and cries out for help.

Here's a little story of an office problem that I use to illustrate the origin of sickness.

Once upon a time, there was a little business which worked in perfect harmony. It made good products, enjoyed a good reputation, and was assured of a good clientele that was more than satisfied and faithful. The company prospered. Everyone knew what they had to do every day. There were no problems and everyone was happy.

One day, the receptionist failed to show up. Everyone else manned the pumps. First one, and then the other, was answering the telephone, opening and distributing the mail, doing the scheduling. Meanwhile, they were still going to business meetings and receiving their own clients. The receptionist failed to show up for work more and more frequently. But nobody really worried because, by now, they were used to it.

Sure, everyone had to take a little more responsibility on their shoulders, but they held the fort. Even though they finished later, arrived home later, and were more and more tired. After a while, they lost their enthusiasm and peace of mind. Their attitude to their clients wasn't the same. They no longer had time to chat with them. But the clients remained faithful and nothing appeared untoward.

But then came the day when the accountant had a car accident and was laid up for a few days. This only added to the problem. Everyone did their best, but they were overloaded, and fell behind. Then the inevitable happened. The director of marketing, who was looking after the accounting temporarily in addition to his other functions, which were already over-loading him, made a mistake in writing out a cheque. Instead of $5,000, he wrote $50,000. In light of such a serious error, he was fired.

After that, things went from bad to worse. Management and staff were simply unable to cope. Mistakes became more and more frequent. Each time, one accused or dismissed the person who had made the mistake, rather than evaluate the situation as a whole and realize that the problems had begun when the receptionist had started failing to show up for work, more and more often. The personnel was exhausted. Clients were dissatisfied with the products and service they were receiving. A short while later, the business closed. It declared bankruptcy.

And yet, the problem was simple. The receptionist was missing work because the woman who had looked after her children while she was at the office had quit. And she had been unable to find a full-time replacement. Rather than punish those who had made mistakes, one only had to identify the receptionist's problem and help her find someone to look after her youngsters. The company would still be in business.

Visible body:
physical

Manifestation
of the problem

Invisible
bodies:
thoughts /
emotions

The problem
itself

Soul:
conscience

Cause of the
problem

The natural order goes:

from the interior to the exterior
from the invisible to the visible
from the depth to the surface
from the cause to the manifestation.

Finding and correcting the cause
of the problem: the soul

If we want to definitely resolve the problem, CURE, then we will have to go beyond the problem itself. More in depth, right to its origin. What is causing the problem? Why is there an iceberg in the first place? Where does it come from? What caused it to arise?

It is the ultimate step in medicine. It is the medicine of the soul. It ascertains that the conscience is sleeping. It awakens it. It alerts the soul, the "raison d'être" of our existence on earth. It asks it the fundamental question:

WHO IS AT THE SERVICE OF WHOM?

Only the soul has the power to choose

- If the soul chooses submission, it is sickness.
- If the soul chooses sovereignty, it is health.
- If the soul does not choose, it chooses submission, by default.

To correct the problem, the soul must:
- pass from the materialistic to the spiritualistic option.
- take a decision and act accordingly.
- for it is in the soul that the conscience (captain, orchestra leader), which decides, resides.

THE SOUL IS SUBMISSIVE

- The naturel order is over-turned.
- The system is upside down.
- The ship is capsized.

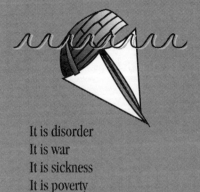

It is disorder
It is war
It is sickness
It is poverty

VICIOUS CIRCLE OF SICKNESS

Submission of the soul permits low vibrations to take over.

Povery and fear take hold.

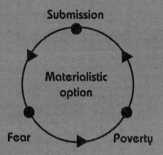

Submission ➡ fear + poverty

IT IS UP TO US TO DECIDE

THE SOUL IS SOVEREIGN

- The natural order is respected.
- The system is as it should be.
- The ship navigates well.

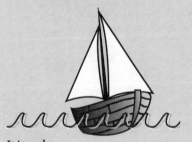

It is order
It is peace
It is health
It is prosperity

HARMONIOUS CIRCLE OF HEALTH

The sovereignty of the soul raises the vibrations of the invisible and visible bodies.

Love and prosperity follow.

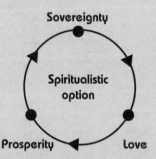

Sovereignty ➡ love + prosperity

VICIOUS CIRCLE OF SICKNESS

The soul is at the service of the body.
The traveller is at the service of the vehicle.
The spirit is at the service of matter.

IT IS THE MATERIALISTIC OPTION

The visible and invisible bodies dominate.
The soul is submissive.
The captain (conscience) remains asleep, drunk, or paralyzed.

To give priority to matter over spirit, is to go against the natural order. It is to go anti-clockwise. It is to give priority to the tip of the iceberg, to that which is visible.

IT IS TO CHOOSE DISORDER, SICKNESS, DEATH

WHO IS AT THE SERVICE OF WHOM?

HARMONIOUS CIRCLE OF HEALTH

The body is at the service of the soul.
The vehicle is at the service of the traveller.
The matter is at the service of the spirit.

IT IS THE SPIRITUALISTIC OPTION

The soul dominates the visible and invisible bodies.
The body follows.
The captain (conscience) awakes and retakes control.

To give priority to spirit over matter, is to go with the natural order, with common sense, clockwise. It is to give priority to the base of the iceberg, to that which is invisible.

IT IS TO CHOOSE ORDER, HEALTH, LIFE

Vicious circle of sickness

Let us see what happens in each of our bodies and in the soul when we live a life that gives priority to the materialistic option. And at the consequences of such a choice.

The major sickness of the soul: submission

It is the prison of the conscience. It locks one up. It renders its victims powerless and unhappy. We submit to the circumstances rather than master them. We sink into lethargy, silence and passiveness. We let others do our thinking for us, and make our decisions theirs. We let fear invade our home and muzzle the conscience.

Submission translates into symptoms of feelings of **powerlessness** and **hopelessness**. Two recognized major causes of cancer and suicide. It feeds the sicknesses of auto-destruction such as drugs, alcoholism, and degenerative illnesses. It robs us of our very essence and our most profound aspirations to improve and do better.

Submission reduces us to a robot, a servile machine, a potentially very profitable commodity. It strips us of our superior functions of consciousness and will. It is a direct attack on our human dignity.

Submission is the major cause of sickness. And yet, our entire system encourages submission. Schools reward quiet children who do as they are told and punish the rebellious. Universities teach uniformity and discourage creativity. The establishment severely punishes those who disobey. There is simply no place for a maverick. The worst form of submission that one can impose upon people is social assistance. And we are all socially assisted. Health insurance, unemployment benefits, life insurance, salary insurance, pension funds, welfare, taxes and others. All these measures to make us dependent upon the authorities. Because we believe that we cannot do it for ourselves. We end up being treated like sheep.

The major sickness of the invisible bodies: fear

Fear of losing what we have. Fear of not having what we want. Fear of the past, the present, and future. Fear of being robbed, raped, condemned, ridiculed. Fear of failure. Fear of losing one's job. Fear of flying. Fear of the dark. Fear is **the basket of all emotions**. It contains them all. Fear paralyzes the conscience. It renders one blind and powerless. Yet fear is on the rise every day in our society what with all its criminality, job losses, bankruptcies, the recession, sickness, wars, and violence. It is enough to make anyone afraid. The media hardly ever seems to mention anything else. Have you heard any good news lately, except in the realm of sports? Apart from artists, who are having a rough time making ends meet, who talks to us of love?

> **"The mass of men lead lives of quiet desperation. What is called RESIGNATION is confirmed DESPERATION."**
>
> Thoreau

And as thought generates reality, therefore, when we hear on the news that four out of ten women will suffer from breast cancer, we think that one of them will be us. And we are afraid. The thought, and the emotion, "cancer" implants itself in our invisible bodies and the cancer will appear in the physical body sooner or later. We have programmed it.

Fear brings sickness. And yet, the powers that be conspire to create it. Fear freezes us and turns our blood to ice. It keeps the icebergs in place. Belief, its twin sister, ravages our thoughts just as much as fear does the emotions. The most deeply rooted belief is that we are not all equal.

The major sickness of the visible body: poverty

Poverty is the **mother of all misfortune**. It gives rise to all calamities. It has been demonstrated a thousand times over that the level of sickness is directly linked to that of poverty. The poor are sick. They all have physical, emotional or social problems. Mothers give birth to small, underweight babies whose health is compromised and mortgaged from the moment they are born and for the rest of their lives. And all it takes is a minimum of good nutrition to ensure the birth of a normal-sized baby and save the economy tens of thousands of dollars in medical costs, both immediate and future. Poverty is the biggest cause of sickness.

It is the vicious circle of sickness.

SUBMISSION ⟶ FEAR ⟶ POVERTY ⟶ SUBMISSION

Harmonious circle of health

Let us see what happens in each of our bodies and in our soul when we live a life that has a spiritualistic priority. And at the consequences of our choice regarding health.

The health of the soul: sovereignty

As a sovereign person, you are the supreme authority of your life. You exercise your inner power rather than submit to the power of the authorities. You are in full control of your thoughts, and emotions. You know no boundaries and are full of creativity.

It is easy to encourage sovereignty among individuals. We only have to remember the divine essence of each and every one of us, for us to realize that "we can do it". And that many people, united and working together, can move mountains. And build a society that is rich and in good health.

The health of the invisible bodies: love

"There are only two emotions: love and fear. The first is our natural heritage. The other, a creation of our spirit." - Jampolsky.

To discourage fear, one only has to stop talking about security and protection, two impracticable illusions. To encourage love, it is sufficient to create links between individuals. To bring them to discover and to get to know one another, like one another, and help one another.

Love is warmth. It has always melted icebergs. Progressively, the symptoms disappear, and then the entire iceberg.

Unfortunately, the authorities promulgate hate, suspicion and distrust. Every man for himself. Nothing that promotes health.

The health of the visible body: prosperity

Individual sovereignty ensures prosperity and abundance for all. Being on the same wavelength as our inner divinity assures us of real and unique security. Namely, assurance, that which no one can take from us and from which flows prosperity, in all its forms:

- **physical:** adequate food and housing, vital and recreational space, pure air and water.
- **psychological:** love, belonging, recognition, consideration in the home, at school, work and at play.
- **spiritual:** dignity, power, identity, passion, respect for one's differences, value in originality and creativity.

It is the harmonious circle of health.

SOVEREIGNTY ➡ LOVE ➡ PROSPERITY ➡ SOVEREIGNTY...

Re-establishing the natural order to go from sickness to health

The deeper the problem, the more fundamental it is. Therefore we have to re-establish the order of priority of our solutions, beginning with those at the deepest level, and working towards those that are the most superficial.

The soul being the deepest, solutions that will improve its state of health are therefore key.

1. This is why the priority action must focus on the sovereignty of the soul (medicine of self-healing).

2. At the same time, we have to make every effort to re-establish the health of the invisible bodies. For us to rid ourselves of the emotions and thoughts which imprison us, and instead spread love and sharing (alternative medicines).

3. And last but not least, we have to take care of our physical body in terms of food, hygiene, non-pollution, and lifestyle.

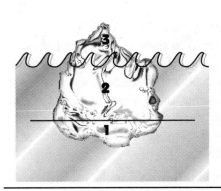

Physical body

Invisible bodies

It is in the inner co[r]
of the hidden part of th[e]
iceberg wherein lie[s]
the root of the proble[m]
that must be cure[d]

Soul

It is obvious that all these different types of medical practices overlap, and that one influences the other. This is why medicine must offer patients different alternatives for the well-being of their bodies and soul. Concomitant treatments touching both medicines and calling upon the skills of doctors and therapists at the same time.

There exists many books which explain, in easy-to-understand terms, the different practices of medicine from self-health to the rarest of illnesses, as well as everything one needs to know about nutrition and all facets of daily hygiene. It is up to us to determine which best suits our needs.

One book that merits special attention is, **Take Charge of Your Body** by Carolyn DeMarco. I highly recommend it to all women and all health practitioners.

And I cannot fail to mention all the books written by Serge Mongeau on medicine and health. **Pour une nouvelle médecine (For a New Medicine)** contains all the elements necessary to expand our knowledge of a true medicine of health.

WHERE SHOULD OUR MONEY GO?

Towards health, because that is our best investment. First of all, to the health of the soul, because it is in the soul that sickness is born... so too is the cure. In practical terms, our money should go first towards education which leads to empowerment.

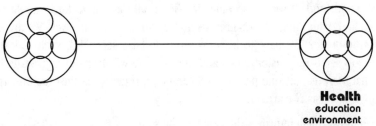

Sickness
scientific medicine

Health
education
environment
alternative medicines
fees
administration

1) To education

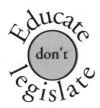

Education brings knowledge. Knowledge is a tool which leads to power. When we know, we control. To educate is to share knowledge. It is to share power. It is empowering others. It is to give information that will enable others to control their health, their life. The education of health is that which makes people aware of their divine and all-powerful nature. It gives us the tool to break free from the illusion of sickness/death and pass on to the reality of health/life. If we are ill, then it is because we have distanced ourselves from our divinity. We only have to come back to it to be healed.

Education leads to empowerment. That is to say, the reinforcement of our inner power. The power OF. We are all-powerful, but we have forgotten it. Education reminds us of this and teaches us how to free ourselves from the ideas that imprison us, notably the illusions that we entertain.

Namely, physical and mental suffering, sickness, aging, death. Education also teaches us how to replace the paralyzing emotion of fear (creation of fear = illusion) with the all-powerful emotion of love (innate = reality). In this way, we will no longer be slaves, but free. We will leave the bleak jungle and enter "the garden of life", as my friend Louise Pomminville would say.

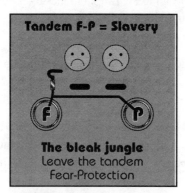

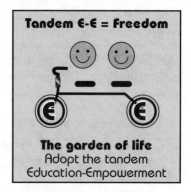

Education enables us to evaluate the **intention** which underpins all politics and decisions. These must be clearly understood so that people can take their rightful place and actively participate in the formulation of decisions.

Schools should encourage creativity and initiative. Painting, drawing, or any other art form helps one to develop ideals. Silence and nature enables one to get one's bearing again and a better perspective on life.

We should learn self-health. How to take charge of our health, learn how to select good food. If we do become sick, learn all there is to know about our illness and, with the help of therapists and doctors, cure ourselves. We are the only true doctor. We have to learn to set aside false securities, such as insurance, job security, pension funds and the like. We will learn to appreciate the fact that there is only one person who can help protect us against the only real enemy that exists. We are our own worst enemy.

Empowerment improves the health of the soul.

EDUCATION DOES NOT COST AN ARM AND A LEG

2) To alternative medicines

As a general rule, remember that chronic illnesses and those which are said to be psychiatric in nature are in the domain of alternative medicines.

They comprise treatments which treat and reinforce, which is real prevention. They free blocked energy, while rebalancing and reinforcing the entire energy system. The role of healers is to be found at this level. They re-establish energy in the invisible bodies and help them to become stronger, as well as replacing the energy, as the case may be. Healers sometimes work with the help of "guides" that are invisible to the majority of us. These are the "doctors of the sky" of whom Maguy Lebrun speaks about in her book **Médecins du ciel, médecins de la terre (Doctors of the Sky, Doctors of the Earth)**. She also explains just how much more powerful the energy of healing is when we work together in a group.

ALTERNATIVE MEDICINES DO NOT COST AN ARM AND A LEG

3) To the environment

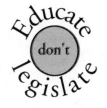

- To take care of Mother Earth, our hostess. To learn how to respect and venerate her. Thank her for having welcomed us. Stop chemically polluting the air, water, and soil. Stop stripping forests and changing the course of our rivers and waterways. Realize that we are at her service, and not she at ours. Our fate depends on her.

- To ensure hygiene for all, having access to clean drinking water, suitable lodging, and a healthy environment. Reduce consumerism and all the waste that this generates. Purify the air in workplaces.

- To provide food that is both physically and mentally nutritious. Produce that has not been bombarded with rays. Encourage biological horticulture and, where possible, community and family gardening.

- Make sports and art activities available to all. Make it easy to go to the country. Take charge of communications and ensure the quality of media information. Replace violence and fear in the print and electronic media with respect for the person and love. Encourage positive thinking.

- Promote simple and extensive public transit systems so as to encourage exchange between individuals.

- Poverty must be eliminated by all means possible. Install an economy of need based on richness for all. We must remember that it is not technology that has prolonged our life span, but rather hygiene, and improvement in the quality of our lives.

The refrigerator has done more for health than open-heart surgery.

Poor people are more ill than rich people. People living in poor countries have a life expectancy well below those of people living in rich countries. The rate of infant mortality is also far greater. Poverty and sickness go hand in hand.

HEALTH OF THE ENVIRONMENT DOES NOT COST AN ARM AND A LEG

4) To cover other costs

- **Professional salaries** which are directly proportional to services we receive, therefore not as high.
- **Administrative costs**, which would also be reduced, as they would relate to a smaller "health machine".

THE MEDICINE OF HEALTH DOES NOT COST AND ARM AND A LEG

And what about scientific medicine?

Is it the end of scientific medicine? Not at all. It will always have its place and we will always have need of doctors that have been trained in science and technology. At the same time, however, they must realize their limits.

- They should only use scientific medicines and drugs when it is not possible to treat the patient by other methods.
- They should learn, but not practice, alternative medicines. For they are incapable. It is contrary to their training.
- They should work together with therapists and patients.

As a general rule, remember that trauma, emergencies, and acute illnesses are those which most often have need of treatment by scientific medicine. But not over extended periods of time. Only for the duration of the acute crisis. Once this has passed, such aggressive treatments must be stopped. In many cases, surgery that is debilitating and expensive can be replaced by a method of treatment that is much simpler and less expensive.

It is the case with heart by-pass operations, for example, which may be replaced by a chelation and costs about $3,000 as opposed to the $50,000 it can cost for the operation. As another general rule, unless there is a real obvious emergency, nothing should be done to upset nature which knows how to take care of itself. *"Step zero, do nothing"*, says Susun Weed in the wise-woman tradition mentioned earlier.

If we learn to adopt this attitude, we will save ourselves a lot of grief. Never resort to the medicine of science for preventative purposes. It is like taking a hammer to kill a fly buzzing around on a window pane. You don't always kill the fly. But you always break the window!

THE MEDICINE OF SICKNESS COSTS AN ARM AND A LEG

HOW MUCH WILL ALL THIS COST?

To reduce the exorbitant cost of our health systems, we must pass from a system of sickness to a system of health. In practice, this implies that we considerably reduce our use of tests and medications, and invest a little of the money saved in health. When I say considerably reduce, I do mean considerably. That is to say, eliminate all tests and medications that are not absolutely necessary and justified. This represents between 75% and 95% of current tests, medications and surgical operations. I can hear you shouting, "but that's crazy, its madness". Well, rest assured, the figures are as high as that. One just has to want it, to transform it into reality.

In years to come, the health of everyone would be greatly improved and costs would be much lower. Even if we only managed to reduce the health costs by 25% in the United States, it would save a whopping $250,000,000,000 (250 billion). That's close to $1,000 for every man, woman and child.

As the chart which follows shows, if we succeeded in going even further than that, the savings become astronomical.

Take, for example, a budget of 1 trillion dollars	
total budget of sickness	$1.000.000.000.000
reduce it by 75%	- $750.000.000.000
balance remaining	= $250.000.000.000
add 25% to health budget	+ $250.000.000.000
total cost of sickness/health	= $500.000.000.000

This represents a saving of close to $2,000 per individual. We can reduce our total costs and have a population that is in far better health. One that will benefit both from state-of-the-art scientific technology and the refinement of alternative medicines. It is the best of both worlds. ***Science and art combined*** at the service of the patient.

The solution is obvious and simple. Anyone can find it. But why isn't it applied?

Why is industry still allowed to pollute the water, the air and foodstuffs?

Why are people still left homeless, hungry, living in slums, or working in unhealthy conditions?

Why is all the emphasis placed on competition, conformity, obedience, submission, fear?

Why is materialism pushed and not spiritualism?

Why do we dwell on the inevitability of aging and death?

Why are alternative medicines ridiculed and forbidden?

Why are vaccinations allowed to continue?

Why are people encouraged to take pills and drugs?

Why is ignorance and dependence promoted? Why?

CONCLUSION

What is happening?

All the information exists, and it has for some time now, to enable the authorities to introduce an effective and less costly medicine of health. They have not done it. Not only have they not done it, but they have done exactly the opposite. They are plunging us even deeper into sickness and submission, a little more each day.

- Budgets for social services such as daycare, battered women, recreational centers, help for single mothers, health associations, etc., are cut.

- The gap between rich and poor continues to widen, even during the 80s when times were said to be good and prosperous. We are all affected by this, we will all be poor if we continue like this. What we often fail to realize is that the rich are now much richer, and there are fewer of them than before.

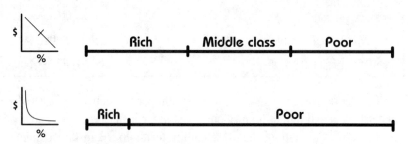

- Concentration of money in the hands of a few;
- Progressive disappearance of the middle class into poverty.

- Welfare dependency in all its forms is increasing everywhere, as is unemployment, people on pensions, and those collecting health insurance. In losing our jobs and becoming poorer, in becoming sick and older, we become to depend upon the State with all the loss of human dignity that this entails.

A thought in passing:

With the advent of feminism and women's liberation, more and more women have been freed from the guardianship of their husbands. They have become autonomous. There are fewer so-called "kept women" than there were one or two generations ago. But, alas! It is now men and women who are being "kept". Not by their wives or husbands but, this time, by the government.

We should always remember that being "kept" is a lousy position to
find oneself in. For even if one has the best "keeper" in the world, one is
always at their mercy, for at any time:

- *they can stop taking care of us, to start taking care of someone else.*

- *or just be simply unable to take care of us any longer.*

In either case, we lose what we have. In all cases, we lose our dignity.
And remember that submission is the basis of all illnesses.

- Industries continue to pollute the air, water, and soil. Every day, we discover
that such and such a region is suffering from some sort of illness directly
related to a polluting industry. And we go on.

For example, many people living around the Great Lakes in both
Canada and the United States suffer from sterility. Rather than resolving the
problem at its source, the problem of pollution, we develop methods of fer-
tility.

- Alternative medicines are banned and those who practice them are hounded.
The authorities harass, threaten, and intimidate them without any reason
whatsoever.

- "Health" insurance, both public and private, reimburses only sickness.
Alternative medicine therapies are not reimbursed at all as they are in some
countries.

- Good remedies are banned. The authorities pass laws declaring them illegal.
They are therefore withdrawn from the market and become inaccessible to
the public at large.

- Everything contributes to creating fear among the public. The media
projects nothing but violence, war, misfortune, sickness and all that this
entails. Recessions, budget cuts, debts, and so on. **Fear is the vehicle of
sickness.**

Why are the political, medical, and financial authorities doing all in their
power to ruin our health and our bank account? Shouldn't the government, our
representative, look after our interests? It is paid for that. Not only is it not doing
so, but it is doing just the opposite. Why? Three hypotheses present themselves:

1st hypothesis:

They do not know how to do it.

This explanation is impossible, because the information has existed for years. *Medical Nemesis - The Expropriation of Health* by Ivan Illich dates from 1975. Some 20 years ago, we were warned of the disastrous consequences that awaited us with the practice of scientific medicine. Since 1980, several books have denounced - and continue to do so - the corruption, yes even the conspiracy, against our health. Several other books have proposed solutions.

Therefore, the government knows the problems that exist and knows how to remedy them.

2nd. hypothesis:

They cannot do it.

This explanation is also impossible, because the government has all the powers. The power to inform, the power to educate, the power to finance, the power to legislate, the power to enact that legislation. It can therefore do anything that it wishes.

3rd. hypothesis:

They do not want to do it.

This explanation is the only one possible, once the other two hypotheses are eliminated. One always thinks that governments, and their civil servants, are without intelligence and really don't put their hearts into their work. How can we be so mistaken. One also always thinks that they act in good faith, but that they are simply overburdened by the amount of work that they have to do. How can we be so mistaken.

"There is none more deaf than those who will not hear". It is true as far as our demands are concerned. We can also add: "There is none more paralyzed than those who wish to maintain the status quo."

The current system of sickness is a disaster for our health and our finances. Moreover, it displeases everyone. However, it must profit someone, if, despite everything, it has been maintained for all these years.

PROFIT WHOM?

The obstacle:
The Medical Mafia

THE REAL BENEFICIARY OF THE MEDICAL SYSTEM

Doctors and patients alike are concerned with health, each from their own perspective. They should be able to reorient themselves and create a more effective health policy.

WHY DON'T THEY DO IT?

Because these two actors in the system have become silent and powerless spectators. They no longer have any power over their health. Nor over its practice. Nor over the financing of health. Who then has taken over this power?

The power of the patients is their financial clout

"He who pays the piper calls the tune", goes the old saying. Well, we have made a lie of that old dictum. Sure, it is the patient who pays. But it is not the patient who calls the tune. It is the **insurance** companies. Whether they are privately-owned or government-run, they take our money and do with it what they think best. As soon as we entrust our money to someone else, we lose the control and freedom to use it as we see fit. They have taken over the stage. And we have relinquished it. We have accepted to sit back and watch the show these actors wish to stage. Whether we like it or not.

The power of the doctors is their knowledge

They place this knowledge at the service of patients who come to consult them. Yet they too have also been dispossessed of their power, reduced to the role of spectators. In effect, doctors do not have free access to medical information, and even less to the practice which seems to them best suited to their patients' needs. Those who decide the practice of medicine are the authorities, the all-powerful medical **institutions**. They have full powers of decision over the practice of doctors. The doctors are their instrument, their means of action. They form and shape them, and keep them in their mold, at their service.

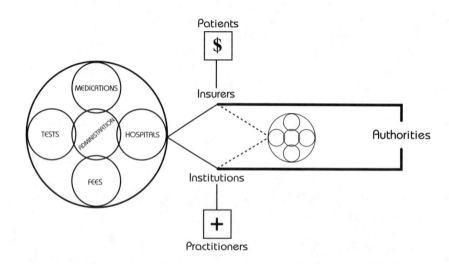

The usurped power of the authorities

The patient and the doctor wish to meet one another to exchange. One, the patient, brings the money ($), the other, the knowledge (+). But the authorities prevent this direct meeting.

authorities
=
insurers
+
institutions

- The insurers, the **financial authority**, deviate the money towards illness.
- The institutions, the **legal authority**, deviate the practice of health towards illness.

Therefore, the patient and doctor can only meet **indirectly**, through the intermediary of the authorities, in the realm of the **illness**. Health is short-circuited and inaccessible.

FINANCIAL POWER + LEGAL POWER = TOTAL POWER

Doctors know only one medicine: sickness. Who goes to see a doctor if they are not sick? Nobody. In addition, patients are not entitled to medical services unless they are sick. No sickness, no medicine. Doctors are not reimbursed for their "health" services. Only for their "sickness" services.

Doctors who stray from the narrow paths that are recognized and approved by the established powers that be pay dearly for it. They are assailed by fear, harassment, intimidation, threats. They are dragged before a disciplinary committee, lose their right to practice, pay fines, are carted off to prison. For some years now, it is a witch-hunt aimed at all health practitioners, whether they be doctors or therapists.

So the two actors of the system, the patient and doctor, have lost their role as actors. But then who has taken their place? Who are the real, true actors?

If we cannot discover who is preventing the actors from playing their roles, let us ask ourselves whose interests are best served in such a case. Who profits from the current system of sickness? Do they perhaps have a vested interest in seeing such a system survive?

Those who realize a profit from the system of sickness are undoubtedly the beneficiaries of the largest sums of money dispensed by the system. And we have already identified the three major expenditures:

"The health of citizens is a commodity which is bought and sold."

François Mitterand
President of France

- tests which make a profit for the technological industry.
- medications which make a profit for the pharmaceutical industry.
- hospitals, pharmacies, laboratories, which make a profit for both the above two industries, as well as a plethora of other small industries.

All of these industries have an obvious interest in sickness and would have everything to fear from a population in good health. Most notably it is the pharmaceutical industry, whose profits are far greater than those of most other industries, that has taken control of medicine. How has it been able to do this? How has it been able to tilt the system in its own favour?

A short quiz

One generally speaks of the medical BODY. Now every system comprises a body and a soul. Therefore, if there is a body, there is also a soul.

WHO IS THE MEDICAL SOUL?

Make your choice.

❏ Laboratories   ❏ Government   ❏ Insurers

❏ Charitable   ❏ High technology   ❏ Medical colleges
  organizations

❏ Clinics   ❏ Pharmacists   ❏ Patient

❏ Medicare   ❏ Surgeons   ❏ Therapists

❏ Medical associations   ❏ Administrators   ❏ Pharmaceutical
                                                    industry

❏ Hospitals   ❏ Ministry of Health   ❏ Universities

❏ Researchers   ❏ Civil servants   ❏ FDA

For the answer, you'll have to read on...

THE TILTING OF THE MEDICAL SYSTEM

The players in the system

In order to be able to reply to this question, let us recap the five different players on the medical stage and their roles.

1) the patient who consults and pays: . . . . .the client

2) the practitioner who advises: . . . . .the consultant

3) hospitals
   clinics
   laboratories
   pharmacies: . . . . .the executants

4) industry which makes the products: . . . . .the manufacturer

5) the authorities: . . . . .the manager

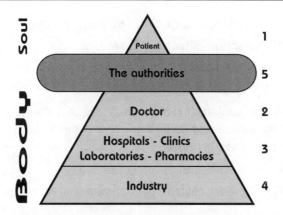

THE SOUL IS THE PATIENT, the essence, the reason for being of the system. Without a soul, there is no body. Without a patient, there is no medical system.

THE BODY IS THE STRUCTURE at the service of the soul. The doctor, hospitals, clinics, laboratories, pharmacies, industry.

All the rest are artificial realizations created to respond to artificially-created needs. The authorities.

Officially

It involves a system of HEALTH at the service of the SOVEREIGN patients. They are the decision-makers, the all-powerful element in the medical system. Officially, they are the supreme authority. The entire health system is at their service. They are its *"raison d'être"*. They are **the SOUL of the system.**

The other players make up the BODY of the system. We spoke earlier of the "medical corps", the "medical body". Strange that we never speak of the "medical soul".

1) PATIENTS: the **clients**. It is they who employ and pay. It is they who have the power of decision.

Their servants

2) DOCTORS: the **consultants**. They are employed and paid. It is they who advise the patients. They are entirely at the patients' service.

3) HOSPITALS, CLINICS, LABORATORIES and PHARMACIES: the **executants**. They are the assistants, dispensors of the services and products deemed necessary for the health of the patient, and complementary to the practice of the doctors:

- **hospitals** which accommodate the very sick and provide very serious forms of treatment.
- **clinics** which dispense lighter forms of treatment and care.
- **diagnostic laboratories** (analyses, X-rays).
- **pharmacies and retailers** which dispense products (medications, glasses, prostheses, etc.).

4) INDUSTRY: **the manufacturers** of goods and products necessary for the health of the patients and doctor's practices in the health system. It is an industry at the service of health:

- **pharmaceutical** which manufactures medications.
- **technological** which manufactures instruments and equipment.

Their managers

5) The AUTHORITIES: the **managers** of the patient. They are the patients' delegates. Their role is to facilitate the medical practice and its administration. It is an artificial creation:

financial
authorities

- the **insurance companies** which "insure the security" of patients. They may be privately- or publicly-owned. In either case, they deduct money from the patient and redistribute it to different players in the medical system which contribute to the good health of the patient.

legal
authorities

- **medical institutions** which "ensure the protection" of patients and doctors. They look after the interests of the public, patients, and doctors. They also control training (faculties, colleges, schools, journals, conventions, teaching), as well as research and publications, the manufacture and authorization of products, grants, fund-raising, institutes and foundations.

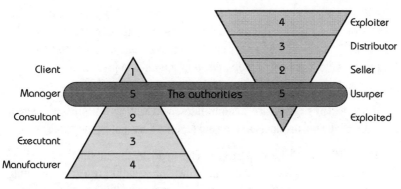

| | **IN THEORY** | | **IN PRACTICE** | |

Health system serving the patient.
The body serving the soul.

Patient at the mercy of a system of
sickness. The soul serving the body.

↓

↓

ORDER
system upright

(DIS)ORDER
System over-turned

**NATURAL ORDER
of divine essence**

**ESTABLISHED ORDER
of the authorities**

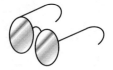

If we take off our rose colored glasses, we perceive quite another scene.
The system is tilted. It is the **patients who are at the service of the system
of sickness**.

The tilting of the system is the result of the intervention by the authorities
who have wedged themselves between the patients and their servants. Without
the intervention of the authorities, who purport to be our agents, there would be
no possible way of tilting the system.

In practice

In this new light, let us look again at the role of each of the players on the
medical stage.

1) PATIENTS: The **exploited** consumers. The more they consume, the better.
   The more sick they are, the more profitable it is. So one has to make sure
   that they are sick. That medications do not cure illnesses. That new illnesses
   are created. The only thing that counts is financial performance as reflected
   on the stock market.

2) DOCTORS: The **sellers**, albeit unaware, of industry. The industry's promotional tools. The authorities form and mold them to serve their goals, blindly,
   faithfully, and to the letter, without ever doubting nor questioning the sanctity
   of the truth. This truth and blind obedience, which the industry commands,
   is set out by the medical establishment.

THE OBSTACLE

It is taught in the form of doctrine to eager medical students who, although full of good intentions, lap it up. After five to ten years of such brainwashing, nobody could fail to succumb. They are also bought with financial privileges and/or steps up the ladder of success. To some, they give prestige. To others power. And to still others they give money. The vast majority are unaware of just how they are being "prepared" for their chosen profession.

3) HOSPITALS, CLINICS, LABORATORIES and PHARMACIES: The manufacturer's **distributors**. They are accomplices who very assiduously convey the manufacturers' products to the patient, for a very handsome profit.

The exploiter is the one who makes an excessive profit from others.

4) The INDUSTRY: The **exploiter**. The head of the medical system. The beneficiary of sickness. Under the cover of scientific research and public concern, it scatters the seeds of sickness and reaps the rewards. With extraordinary tact and diplomacy, it pulls all the strings of the system in the direction it wants it to go and in its own interest. It works in the shadows and through go-betweens. It controls every facet of medicine. From the medical student right up to the patient, which it solicits directly through the media.

The usurper is the one who seizes by unjust means.

No doors are closed to it. All levels of the "authorities", whether they be government or medical, are subject to its immense **power**. After all, it is the industry that has allowed them to rise to power and recognition. All that it asks is that they remember and that they do not bite the hand that feeds them. It rules. Sometimes benignly by corruption. Sometimes dictatorily by fear, threats and punishment. Industry has succeeded in appropriating our supreme Authority. It is an insidious "coup d'état"!

5) The AUTHORITIES: The **usurper**. They have created the institutions and the laws in order to dispossess the patients of their financial and legitimate rights over their health and appropriate these for themselves. They have stripped the patients of their legitimate Authority and replaced it by "authorities" that they legally established.

• divine Authority • innate in everyone • legitimate • illegal	• the authorities • established by force • illegitimate • legal

The impostor is the one who deceives by false appearances, by lies, particularly in passing himself off for someone that he isn't.

In order not to arouse suspicion, the industry has erected a screen. That screen is the GOVERNMENT. This **impostor** with all the airs of a saint coming to our aid, has betrayed us for the sake of profit for the industry. It is elected by us. It is paid by us. But it has sold us off to the industry. Government and its agencies are on the payroll of the industry. The latter finances them and grants them rights of authority over the other players.

Hidden behind yet another screen, this time the veil of government, are its agencies, the insurance companies and the medical institutions.

Globally, they are called "the authorities" and they are revered. They are accorded enormous power. This power, established by the industry, is referred to as the "establishment". Elected politicians and civil servants, whom they will keep just as long as they follow the rules of the game dictated by their superiors, the industry. Should they show the least sign of defiance or waver in their loyalty, they will fall from grace and be cast out. Thanks to government, insurance companies control the money and the institutions, the practice of medicine.

THE ESTABLISHMENT

According to the dictionary, the establishment is *"a powerful group of well-placed individuals who defend their privileges: the established order"*.

The established order versus the natural order

Why has an order been established? Wasn't there one already? Does nature really need to be told what to do? Do flowers wait to be computer-programmed in order to know when they should bloom and wilt? Must we instruct our stomach when to begin digesting food that we have eaten? No. NATURE KNOWS. It follows an order. Its own, **inner**, natural order.

The natural order is inherent in every human being, plant or creature. It is innate. We come into the world with it. Nature, whether it be a person, an animal, or a plant, follows the natural order. And all goes well. It does not need to be told what to do, and has even less need of having this imposed upon it. Flowers grow in spring and die in the fall. Our organism functions harmoniously. The captain of every human being is in command and steers in the right direction, using the waves, wind, currents, as allies. There is peace and health aboard. It is the order.

THE SOUL HAS PRIORITY OVER THE BODY

The established order has come to supplant the natural order. It is acquired. It is imposed by force and violence. The established order puts its pawns in place - the authorities - and gives them power over others, who in turn have to obey.

It makes its own laws and imposes them through tribunals, the police, the army. It goes contrary to nature and the natural law. It must therefore use force to achieve it. It has taken over control from the captain. And so the wind, waves and currents have become foes. And so it is war and sickness. It is DISorder.

THE BODY HAS PRIORITY OVER THE SOUL

Who has established the established order... and for whom?

- The establishment

And who profits from the established order?

- The privileged.

The natural order is innate, every person is his or her **own authority**. Nobody can dominate or exploit the other. Each is in possession of the supreme Authority. Each is sovereign and follows the divine Universal Law, the law which upholds the natural order.	The established order replaces the innate Authority of each individual through **external authorities**, which it names and imposes. As a result, it can dominate and exploit others. Each human being is subjected to, and forced to obey, their laws, laws which ensure the established DISorder.

The power of the privileged

The establishment is a parallel power, contrary to nature, established and imposed by the privileged in order to maintain their privileges.

IT IS A MAFIA

The medical establishment is a parallel medical power, which goes contrary to the power of natural healing. It is established and imposed by the privileged to dominate and exploit the patients and, therefore, maintain the privileges of the privileged.

IT IS THE MEDICAL MAFIA

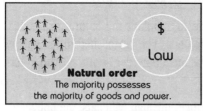

Natural order
The majority possesses
the majority of goods and power.

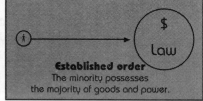

Established order
The minority possesses
the majority of goods and power.

The medical establishment and its associates

The establishment does not only exist in the medical world. It exists in all systems. The political establishment, financial establishment, religious establishment, university establishment, the communications establishment, agro-food establishment, educational establishment, artistic establishment, sports establishment, and so on, and so on. **Privileged people who band together to maintain their privileges.**

All these privileged people pull the strings. There is strength in unity. Make no mistake. All, regardless of what profession or business they are in, are on friendly terms. Even if they do argue sometimes. They help one another, they combine their efforts for but one common objective. To dominate and exploit. It is the **alliance** of power.

IT IS THE ALLIANCE OF MAFIAS

The world medical establishment

The establishment is not only national. Over and above the health system of each country, there exists a world health system. The World Health Organization (W.H.O.), which establishes world health policies. It imposes them progressively on the governments of all countries. It is the globalization of powers.

> **Murder by Injection**
> Eustace Mullins

IT IS THE MAFIA OF MAFIAS

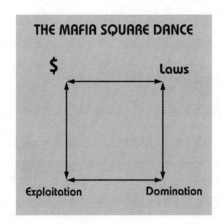

THE MAFIA SQUARE DANCE

$ — Laws

Exploitation — Domination

AUTHORITIES = MAFIA = ESTABLISHMENT

The mafia

A mafia, by definition, is a parallel power, with its own laws, its own justice. But parallel to what? Parallel to whom? Unquestionably, parallel to the official government. But then why does the Mafia enjoy the protection of those in power, the financial and political authorities?

Perhaps it is because the government is also a mafia. And that, as Olivia Zemor reports in her book entitled **The Mafia Above All Suspicion**: "Between honest people, there is always a way to get along." The Mafia-government tandem is as old as the world and it continues today.

The first wants money, the other power. So an exchange is worked out. "You give me this, I'll give you that. And everyone will be happy." If not, it is war. The weapon of government is the law. The weapon of the Mafia is money. Both are based on force and fear. The government comes across as an angel, the Mafia, the devil. Both usurp sovereign power. And they both know it.

If we reflect on what a government actually is, we quickly realize that it is merely a small minority of privileged people who have appropriated the decisional, financial, and judiciary power of the majority. They have stolen our freedom. With our consent, on top of everything else! They have done it with style by making us believe that it was in our own best interest. For our own security and protection. Protection from whom?

THE GOVERNMENT IS THE #1 MAFIA

We call that democracy. We firmly believe that we have the final decisional power as a result of universal suffrage. It consists of putting an X every few years beside one of the names already chosen by the establishment. Let us recognize our tyrants for what they are and who they represent when we exercise our democratic prerogative. Exploitation and domination of the majority by the minority.

AUTHORITIES = MAFIA = ESTABLISHMENT

A FAMILY PORTRAIT

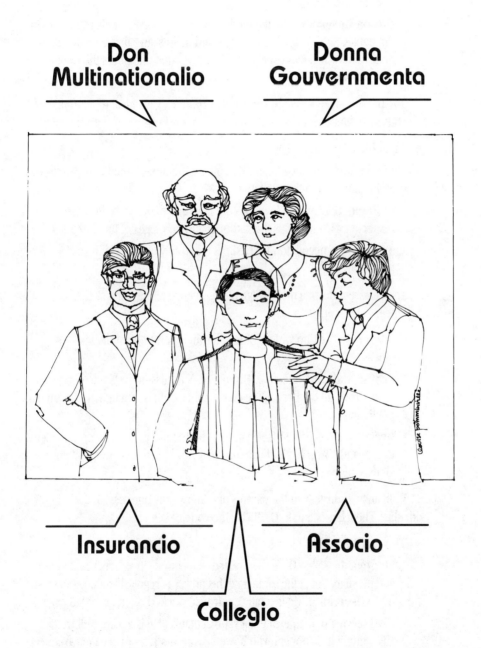

THE MEDICAL MAFIA

Its composition*

- **The parents:** A strong couple. Accomplices for a long time, they have one goal: **the total power of the Godfather**.
  - **Don Multinationalio**, the Godfather, the industry, the purveyor and decision-maker.
  - **Donna Governmenta**, the mother, the government. She is in charge of the house. She establishes the rules and makes sure that everyone does their homework. Everyone takes her for a saint. She obeys the Godfather and serves his interests.

The parents sleep together. Donna Governmenta gave birth to a number of children who the couple needs to run the many facets of the family business.

- **The children:** The TRIO.
  - **Insurancio**, the accountant. He collects the money, public or private, and channels it to the Godfather.
  - **Collegio**, the lawyer. He makes the laws and makes sure they are respected. He maintains the authority and privileges of the Godfather.
  - **Associo**, the negotiator. He ensures the loyalty of the "employees" to the parents.

The children, despite their frequent arguments, all have the same allegiance: to the Godfather.

- **Confidants:** The duo which looks after the operations of the family's business.
  - **Propaganda**, the informer. He ensures submission by gentle persuasion. He controls all the brains, the conventions, courts, scientific publications, publicity, etc.
  - **Gestapo**, the enforcer. He ensures submission by force. He complements Propaganda, with his judiciary machine, and his police, to crush any and all dissenters.

Both answer directly to the parents and know only one master, the Godfather. Their law is harsh: OMERTA, the code of silence.

- **The employees:** Those who faithfully execute all orders.
  - **Medico**, the seller. He is well treated. His complicity is bought with money and prestige. But at the same time, his power is regularly reduced in favour of **Civilservanto**. He is totally controlled, locked up in an gilded cage.
  - **Civilservanto**, the permanent representative. He is always well treated. His complicity is bought with power - over Medico - hence their frequent arguments. Their ongoing rivalry is encouraged.

- **Scientifico**, the researcher. He too is well treated. He collaborates through fraud, conflicts of interest, compromise, political influence, falsification of data. In exchange, he is furnished with laboratory equipment and material, research funds, perks, trips and prestige.

- **The products:** Sold by the family.
  - **Medicamenta**, for chronic and repetitive use.
  - **Surgerica**, for immediate use. May be repeated if need be.
  - **Testa**, for constant use. Before, during, and after the first two.

- **The market:** Targeted by the family.
  - **Patienta**, the commodity to be exploited.
    Generosa, the charitable one. She is mandated to collect as much money as possible from Patienta, to better exploit Patienta.

- **The established rule:** Enforced by the family.
  - **Omerta**, code of silence. No silence, no Mafia.

How it works

Under a health system, which seems incomprehensible because it is so complicated, hides a hierarchy that is extremely simple and harsh. The Godfather reigns supreme. Each family member has a specific function, defined and commanded by the Godfather. Behind the veil of government, industry pulls the strings for its own profit. If the industry were to openly control the medical system, it would run into insurmountable opposition.

We have given up control over our health and our money in accepting to delegate our sovereignty as patients to the authorities. Let us recognize that that, in essence, is the grand art of the impostor on the part of the government and usurpation on the part of industry.

The government

The great impostor. Some of its members realize it, others do not. But all wish to hang on to their position of power. None of them will give up that power lightly, without being forced to, or by becoming aware of the deadly consequences of the system of power.

...and its bodies

The tools of government. At the very top, sit those who ensure government control over the entire health field. Legislative control, financial control, administrative control. It is the State which decides in which major directions the health field will go and what major orientations it will adopt. It controls research and teaching. It decides who will do what, how, when, and where. It controls health and sickness. It exercises its control through the TRIO OF MEDICAL AUTHORITIES.

1) **Insurancio: Health-insurance.** It is the group which manages the patients' money:

   Public, it is Medicare and Medicaid (USA), Health Insurance (Canada), SECU (France). All report to government.

   Private, comprise insurance companies, PPOs, HMOs. They are dependent upon employers and unions. They are regulated by government.

2) **Collegio: The Board/College of Physicians** (L'Ordre des médecins - France, The Board of Physicians - USA, The College of Physicians - Canada). It is an organization of doctors, subsidized by doctors, to protect the public. It is also dependent, in the last instance, upon government. It controls teaching, and issues diplomas. It regulates the right of doctors to practice, and all facets of the medical profession. It may rescind the right of doctors to practice and bar them. It may pursue in court any

   "non-doctor" who opens for business in the health field, citing the illegal practice of medicine. And it is this organization that defines what is medical and what is not! All the power it enjoys has been attributed to it in the name of protecting the public. That is to say for our own good! In reality, it has usurped our right to freedom of choice as sovereign patients, who alone have the right to choose the medicine that best suits us.

3) **Associo: Doctors' Associations.** These too are financed by doctors. But, this time, to protect the interests of doctors. It is these associations that represent doctors in their negotiations with insurance companies for the attribution and allocation of the moneys for medical activities. They are the official spokespersons for doctors. In France, they have very little power. In Canada, not much either. But in the USA, they are very strong. The all-powerful American Medical Association (AMA) that has enormous financial and political clout. It is the second biggest lobbyist after the National Rifle Association (NRA). It benefits from a long tradition of power which dates back to the beginning of the century. And this power has remained very strong ever since. As for France and Canada, it is the College of Physicians and not the associations, which reigns supreme.

All the other medical institutions: control of medications, drugs and instruments (FDA in the United States, Health and Welfare in Canada, Contrôle des médicaments in France); medical schools, research, hospitals, foundations, fund-raising, etc., are dependent upon one or another of the TRIO of medical authorities.

The TRIO

These three large institutions have interests that are very divergent. That is reassuring. It means we can be assured that our interests will be well looked after and defended. Officially, Medicare/Insurance companies assure our interests, taxpayers and consumers. The College/Board defends our interests, the public. The Medical Association defends their interests, the doctors. It is a good war. Two institutions out of three watch over the health and finances of the population. We are in good hands. We can sleep soundly at night.

Wake up! The three institutions are SIBLINGS, born of the same mother, Donna Governmenta, under the control of the same father, the Godfather. Officially, they are three separate entities each with their own address. In reality, they are all fed by the same hand.

Insurancio, Collegio and Associo, while they do not share the same roof, all eat at the same table. As is the case with any family, they argue frequently. More often than not, two children gang up against the third. It is not always the same two. They barter and trade a lot. For example, you pass my law and I'll put a ceiling on doctors' billing rates. Why is it so? Because just like politicians and civil servants, doctors highly placed in these institutions are more concerned with accumulating power than they are about serving other doctors or the patient. And that, the industry has well understood.

Tell me who pays you and I will tell you who you serve

Using its financial power, industry ensures the authority of the government which, in return, ensures its financial interests. I can see you grimacing. I know just how you feel and I agree with you. It is very unsettling to learn that one is being betrayed by the very people in whom one placed all one's trust and confidence. But do we want to keep sticking our head in the sand like an ostrich?

$ ⟷ LAW

The family game of monopoly

The saga of acupuncture

In order to familiarize ourselves with the tactics of the Medical Mafia, let me recount the story of the family's take-over practices in the case of one alternative medicine. The birth, survival, and elimination of acupuncture* in the Province of Québec, Canada. A telling example of what happens in every country where the game is played.

As events unfold, we will be able to observe that the pattern is always the same when it comes to something that could do us some good. Either it is simply outlawed, or it is allowed to slip quietly under the control of the authorities to make it a tool of the medicine of sickness.

The fate of acupuncture is that of almost all alternative medicines, of all natural therapies. It happens in the USA as elsewhere because we, patients, doctors and therapists always make the same mistake. By understanding the tactics of the authorities, let us identify our mistakes, and make sure that we do not make them again.

Let us watch the game unfold!

* Acupuncture is a medical treatment of Chinese origin which consists of using needles to stimulate certain points of the body along vital energy lines. Acupuncture is part of health medicine. It treats the invisible bodies. It re-establishes energy flow and improves health.

DATES	EVENTS
1951	Birth of acupuncture in Québec with the arrival of Oscar Wexu, professor of Chinese acupuncture. Private practice, free of all control by the authorities: • practitioners sell their services • patients buy them • without any law, nor government interference.
1951-1970	Growing popularity of acupuncture. Proportionate growth in client satisfaction.
1968	Beginning of pressure against acupuncture practitioners by the CPMQ (Corporation professionnelle des médecins du Québec). (College of Physicians/Medical Board). Accusation: acupuncturists are charlatans despite the fact clients are very satisfied.
1970	Founding of a private acupuncture school, free of all controls from the authorities. • teachers sell their courses. • students buy them. • without any law, nor government interference.
1970-1977	Acupuncture continues to increase in popularity. As does satisfaction on the part of patients.
1974	Creation of the Office of Professions by the government. It is the new "head" for the "protection of the public". It defines the sector of activity of each profession. It limits professional practice, until now unlimited. It gives **full powers to scientific medicine** over the practice of health, including childbirth (Article 31 of the Medical Law). It also gives scientific medicine the exclusive right to open new specialties in the health field (Article 94 of the Code of Professions).
1977	The CPMQ recognizes the effectiveness and validity of acupuncture and thus **takes over the control** of acupuncture, despite the fact that it knows almost next to nothing about it.
1977-1985	Acupuncture has never been more popular. Patients, who have had access to it and benefited from its therapeutic results, have never been more satisfied.

THE GAME	THE SCORE
Patient Practitioner: acupuncturist More patients More practitioners There are only two actors.	Patients content Practitioners happy
Don Multinationalio frowns. The authorities begin to be worried.	The patient-practitioner partnership works very well.
Don Multinationalio loses patience. **Collegio** = CPMQ begins the witch-hunt. Abuse of power. There is now **1** player of the Mafia.	The liberty of the practitioner is threatened.
Don Multinationalio is angry.	
Donna Governmenta intervenes. She establishes order through legislation. She usurps the rights of patients and practitioners. She collaborates with **Collegio**. There are now **2** players of the Mafia.	Freedom of choice of the patient and the practice of the practitioner limited by the laws and regulations of **- Donna Governmenta** **- Collegio** to "protect the public". True acupuncturists number approximately 800.
Collegio usurps the rights of acupunctur- ists to "protect the public".	
Don Multinationalio orders that it ceases.	The patient-practitioner partnership is undermined.

DATE	EVENTS
July 1985	The CPMQ exercises its control over acupuncture. It passes a regulation that separates the doctor acupuncturists and the "non-doctor" acupuncturists.

The CPMQ exercises its control over acupuncture.
It passes a regulation that separates the doctor acupuncturists and the "non-doctor" acupuncturists.

- Doctors who know nothing about philosophy and the practice of acupuncture, who do not have a clue about energetic medicine, are accorded unfair privileges.

- "Non-doctors" are threatened with prosecution, ordered to retake courses, useless examinations under the control of doctors, and made to incur unjustified expenses to update their skills in order to continue to be allowed to practice.

All to discourage the true acupuncturists and cause them to give up their profession.

DOCTORS	NON-DOCTORS
Right to practice in acupuncture	
Without training, except for 300 hours attending passive theory.	After training of 1,000 hours, theory and practical, in a recognized school.
Inscription in the Registry of Acupuncturists of the CPMQ	
Non-mandatory because already registered.	Mandatory and exacting: conditional upon passing a written and oral exam determined by the CPMQ. Costly: $425 + $200 for each additional entry.
Rules regarding the practice of acupuncture	
Exempted.	Obligated to obtain a medical certificate and provide a treatment report.

DATE	EVENTS
1985	The CPMQ decides to recognize only one new experimental school of acupuncture that is part of the public network that it controls. In doing so, it eliminates the three experienced school of acupuncture, which are forced to close.
1985-1987	The acupuncturists organize themselves, some in associations, others join a union to defend themselves. They are accepted by private insurance companies for the reimbursement of acupuncture treatments. But, on the recommendation of the CPMQ the insurance companies only reimburse treatments dispensed by acupuncturists listed in the Registry, as **"being in good standing"**.

THE GAME	THE SCORE
Collegio deploys his strong-arm tactics: • divide to conquer • abuse of power • legislate outside his field of knowledge • penalize the rebellious acupuncturists • prevent patients from having access to alternative medicines • swing the practice to doctors • ensure the interests of **Don Multinationalio**.	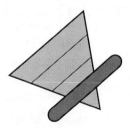 **Collegio** increases his control to the detriment of patient and practitioner. The patient-practitioner partnership is about to disappear.
The doctor, who is the most uninformed and the most ignorant about acupuncture, is favoured over the true acupuncture practitioner. The true acupuncturists are penalized and discouraged in their practice and must submit to all kinds of pressures. Patients who want true acupuncture are discouraged by first having to go and see a doctor, obtain a medical certificate, and pay \$20 to \$100. They are also penalized in this way.	Acupuncture is: 1. in the hands of the authorities who are interested in destroying and misrepresenting it. 2. practiced by greedy doctors who have no other interest in acupuncture but to profit from it. 3. taken from the hands of true acupuncturists. 4. rendered inaccessible to patients by red tape and added costs. 5. changed. Its very essence is altered.
Collegio and **Donna Governmenta** combine their efforts to take control over training in acupuncture. (See the Flexner Report).	Once again, acupuncture sees its quality deteriorate and its essence undermined. The authorities want to replace acupuncture with an acupunctural technique.
New decisions: **Associo**, a new player, positions himself between the acupuncturists and the authorities. **Insurancio**, another new player, places himself between the acupuncturists and the patients and collaborates with **Collegio**. There are now **4** players of the Mafia.	The authorities increase their control to the detriment of patient and practitioner. The patient-practitioner partnership is eliminated.

DATES	EVENTS
1985-1991	The acupuncturists, respecting their true practice, refuse to submit to the medical authorities. - they do not become listed in the Registry. - they do not demand the mandatory medical certificate. And they continue to treat their patients as before. The CPMQ pursues them for "the illegal practice of medicine". It sends bogus patients to visit the insubordinate acupuncturists. Informants paid to trump-up complaints. Because the "real" patients are happy and satisfied. They have no complaints. The acupuncturists have to defend themselves on an individual basis at their own expense. They are forbidden from joining in a class action.
May 1990	By decree, without any justification, the CPMQ lifts their demand that patients should present a medical certificate.
1991	The CPMQ steps up and expands its pursuit against all therapists practicing alternative medicines. The witch-hunt is in full swing.
November 1991	The CPMQ wins its court case against the insubordinate acupuncturists. They are found guilty for having refused to submit to medical domination. As a result, the CPMQ, which knows nothing about acupuncture, is now recognized by the governmental judiciary authorities as having control over acupuncture.
December 1991	The CPMQ proposes and ratifies the signature of an agreement between a group of acupuncturists, their union, and the CPMQ. **The acupuncturists, discouraged and broken, accept the inevitable:** 1) pleading guilty to having practiced acupuncture and renouncing their right to practice. 2) abandoning their right to contest the unjustified lawsuit. 3) restricting the teaching of acupuncture to the only institution designated, and controlled, by the government. 4) submitting to the medical domination and accepting to pass acupuncture exams organized by the CPMQ. 5) inscribing in the CPMQ Registry and paying the enormous costs that this entails. **The CPMQ promises the acupuncturists:** 1) amnesty from all accusations - except one - made unjustly against them by the bogus patients. 2) its "support" in the setting up of their own Corporation, one that would be autonomous and based on a format of their own choosing. The acupuncturists, therefore, were hoping that they would at least be free, once and for all, from the domination of medical authorities who knew nothing about their field. Yet the CPMQ had made promises to the acupuncturists that exceeded their jurisdiction. Moreover, these promises so angered the president of the Office of Professions and the responsible government minister. The revenge was not long in coming.

THE GAME	THE SCORE
Collegio decrees that the acupuncturists are guilty of "the illegal practice of medicine" and pursues them in the courts. **Donna Governmenta** places her judiciary machine at the disposal of **Collegio** to squelch the insubordinate acupuncturists, and accepts the false testimony of bogus witnesses in denouncing the illegal practices.	The acupuncturists are exhausted. Physically, mentally, and financially. 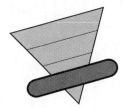
Collegio changes the rules to suit his own ends.	
Collaboration between **Collegio** and **Donna Governmenta/Justicia** to put down and control the true acupuncturists who work to improve health.	The acupuncturists are deceived, harassed, and then crushed. They had believed in justice and democracy and they have been had.

Divide and conquer

Complicity between **Collegio** and **Associo** to deceive the acupuncturists and get them to sign a fraudulent agreement. Complicity between **Collegio** and **Governmenta/Educatio** to recuperate university training in acupuncture for their doctor members.	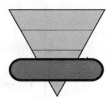

The death of acupuncture

The acupuncturists are made to accept the arrival of a new player, The Office of Professions, an offspring of **Donna Governmenta**, in order to obtain their own Corporation and free themselves from the domination of **Collegio**. There are now **7** players of the Mafia.	The acupuncturists are eliminated from the game. Only 200 survive. Acupuncture is placed under medical domination. The interest of patients is of no importance whatsoever.

DATES	EVENTS
March 1992	The president of the Office of Professions takes everyone by surprise by submitting a bill to Parliament on acupuncture. This document, written in the heat of anger, intended to annul and reverse the promises made by the CPMQ to acupuncturists.
Since March 1992	The union, to which acupuncturists belong, continues to have its members believe that the terms of the agreement with the CPMQ (which it recommended) will eventually be respected by the Office of Professions. Even though the union was aware that the president of the Office of Professions had declared that no part of his proposed bill was negotiable.
June 17, 1994	Bill 34 is passed. This "Law on Acupuncture" creates a Corporation of Acupuncture to govern the practice of acupuncture for "non-doctor" acupuncturists. It does not apply to doctor acupuncturists. In effect, Bill 34: 1) Makes acupuncture a practice of "needle-therapy". It reduces the true practice of acupuncture from one of holistic medicine to that of a simple "pain-killer" technique. 2) Forces patients to first run the medical gauntlet before having access, in the last instance, to acupuncture. 3) Transforms a medicine of health into a medicine of sickness. 4) Places "non-doctor" acupuncturists under government jurisdiction. 5) Favours inept doctors to practice acupuncture to the detriment of those who are true acupuncturists. 6) Creates a number of different types of acupuncture, which does nothing but confuse the patients.

THE GAME	THE SCORE
A cock fight between **Collegio** and **Donna Governmenta/Office of Professions. Donna Governmenta** gets her revenge and has shown her authority over **Collegio** to the detriment of acupuncturists and, above all, over the public who ends up the big loser.	Acupuncturists are now become mere technicians performing "needle-therapy".
The complicity continues between **Collegio** and **Associo** to shut out the duped acupuncturists. The dice are cast. **Donna Governmenta** and her children, **Collegio**, **Insurancio**, and **Associo** return quietly home and tell **Don Multinationalio** that the mission is accomplished. Acupuncture can no longer threaten his pharmaceutical interests. **Don Multinationalio** congratulates them and promises not to forget them!	Acupuncture is finally recuperated by the authorities: - genuine acupuncture has been eliminated - true acupuncturists are handcuffed - doctor acupuncturists are free to do as they wish - new acupuncturists are "trained" in the science of acupuncture in the new schools set up by the authorities - patients become more and more dissatisfied.
Don Multinationalio has won: to all intents and purposes, acupuncture is under his control.	Acupuncture is now a medicine of sickness under the control of the authorities.

The tactics of the Mafia are always the same

1. **Look after** the interests of **Don Multinationalio** and do nothing as long as he is not threatened.

2. **Ban**, any therapy, person, or product that threatens the profits of **Don Multinationalio**, because it will improve health, in the name of charlatanism, and "for the protection of the public". Begin the witch-hunt. **Don Multinationalio** adroitly manipulates the legal system by getting **Donna Governmenta** to protect his interest with our money.

3. **Recuperate,** if these steps are not enough to stop competition, in order to control. Charlatanism of yesterday becomes a blessing of today. Under the protection of the Medical Mafia.

4. **Push** the therapy towards a more scientific technological bent by controlling the training and the functioning of the practice. It also determines the "official" remuneration.

The weapons of the Mafia are always the same

1. **Divide** to conquer. The end justifies the means.

2. **Enact laws.** They can always be amended, changed, or modified, according to its needs.

3. **Complicate** the system and its vocabulary (technocratic jargon) so that the public cannot understand anything. Complicate the means of access to the therapy so as to discourage those who wish to benefit from it.

4. **Crush** the rebels by all methods possible. First, declare them illegal and eliminate then. Then later, legalize them, integrate them, and control them.

The mistakes of practitioners are always the same

1. **Competing with one another** instead of working together. Judging other practitioners and setting up self-serving groups and associations. Encroaching on each other's fields.

2. **Fighting with the Mafia**. Be it in attack, or defense, it is nothing but a war game. It leads to a series of battles, primarily legal, in which the Medical Mafia is always victorious. It controls the laws, as well as the judicial machinery. It is always a no-win situation.

3. **Asking to be recognized by the authorities.** With diplomas, endorsements, approvals, professional corporations, associations, schools, etc. It is giving someone else the power to judge. It is to give up power to others. It is forgetting that

> **AUTHORITIES = MAFIA = ESTABLISHMENT**

Letting even one member of the Mafia come between the patient and the practitioner, for whatever reason whatsoever, is always the beginning of the end of a death knell to a sane patient-practitioner partnership.

4. **Dealing with the Mafia**: **Associo, Collegio, Insurancio, Donna Governmenta,** and all their bodies. It is forgetting that they are all in the pay of **Don Multinationalio** and that:

- the only masters to be served are the sovereign-patients.
- the only allies are the journalists. Inform them continuously.

The mistakes of the patients are always the same

1. Ensuring their **protection** by relying on the authorities' seal of approval.
2. Ensuring their **security** by entrusting it to the insurance companies.
3. **Believing in the authorities** and following their directives.
4. **Believing more in titles and diplomas** rather than in their own sound judgement. For example, believing that doctors are better than therapists is forgetting that common sense is not learned in a classroom.

Let us learn from our mistakes

1. **By exercising our sovereignty as patients**. Complete and exclusive control over the practice of our health and its financing.
2. **By establishing an exclusive patient-practitioner partnership**. One that is closely knit with nobody in between. Assure the practitioner of our full support in the case of an attack by the Medical Mafia. And put it in writing.

Let us join forces together as sovereigns

- Complementary **patient-therapist-doctor** groups sitting around the same table for the management of our health.
- **Patient-consumer-journalist** groups for the realization of our health rights and freedom of choice. Not falling into the same old trap of "putting pressure on government to obtain these". We have nothing to gain, even less to demand, nor do we need their recognition. We have all the rights. We are sovereign. Let us all recognize this and exercise these rights. And watch out anyone who wants to prevent us from doing so!
- **Patient-journalist-practitioner** groups to gather and spread real and truthful information, not that which is filtered down or biased. These groups could organize medical conventions, financed and orchestrated by a committee mandated by them.
- **Patient-patient-practitioner** groups for practicing together the art of living and coming to the aid of those less fortunate. Helping to support them morally and financially until they recover their health and prosperity.

Dear ....,

I appreciate being able to count on you for my health. Yet I am aware that this does represent some risk to you and I thank you for doing it all the same.

I want you to know that you can count on my entire collaboration and support at any time. I am at your disposal. You only have to call.

Your supporter

The couple
Don Multinationalio-Donna Governmenta

The "industrial-governmental complex"

It is always present in whatever system one studies. Sometimes it is subtle. Other times more obvious. The couple is the corner-stone of every Mafia. There are no single-parent families in the Mafia. The **Don** provides the money to get **Donna** elected. She, in turn, passes the laws necessary to ensure profits for the **Don**. For centuries, money and power have always made for good bedfellows. They are inexorably intertwined. Always close by the couple are the children and other players, the accomplices necessary for the success of the operations. They each specialize in a certain field of activities.

- In the MEDICAL field, Carter described it well in his book **_Racketeering in Medicine_**. He calls it the "medico-pharmaceutico-industrial complex". It is organized medicine. Already, in 1984, Stanley Wohl warned us of an unsuitable marriage in his book **_The Medical Industrial Complex_**.

- In the ARMAMENT field, Pierre Marion, former chief of the French Secret Service, explains in detail the "militaro-industrial complex" in his book **_Le pouvoir sans visage (The Faceless Power)_**. He shows how private interests decide the defense and armament policies of a country.

- In the field of AGRICULTURE, Brewster Kneen made the same "exposé" in **_From Land to Mouth_** . In France, Jean-Clair Dausnes shows how banks and industry have assassinated agriculture.

- What can one say of the most lucrative industry of all, the DRUG industry? It is thanks to the collaboration of government in all countries that the market can flourish so well and make such huge profits. The book **_Dope Inc._**, teaches us all we need to know on this business that is controlled by some of the most respected names in the world. There has never been any intention of stopping this market. The so called *War On Drugs* is one big lie, just as big as that of the *War On Cancer*.

The situation is identical in all fields. You will find a list of books that might interest you in this regard later in these pages.

In addition to the couple's marriage, revealed in the above works, the liaison is there to see with our very own eyes. For one even sees television cereal ads sponsored jointly by a cereal maker and the Ministry of Health! Difficult to miss. What else must they do to make us open our eyes?

W.H.O. - The **Donna** of all **Donnas**

This same industry-government liaison is to be found at the world level. It is the product of the world government, the United Nations. At this level we find **Don Financio,** the world financier Godfather, who invests in the field of health, among others, to make profit. His credo is the following:

THE MORE PATIENTS THERE ARE
THE MORE OFTEN THEY ARE SICK
THE LONGER THEY ARE SICK
THE MORE IT PAYS!

To achieve this even faster, he poisons foodstuffs (agro-food). And pollutes the soil, the water, and the air (chemical industries).

W.H.O. (WORLD HEALTH ORGANIZATION)

She is the world's Ministry of Health. She is married to **Don Financio**. Her allegiance to him is unwavering. Like all good mothers, she passes for a good person, concerned for the well-being of us all. She defines health as a "state of physical, mental and social well-being." She gives the impression of being above all the pettiness and narrow-mindedness of national governments. She recognizes the importance of the mental and social aspects of health. She supports alternative medicines. But, if we look really closely, we realize that health for all, according to W.H.O., means medicalization and vaccinations for all. That is to say, **sickness for all.**

Meet Mr. Smith

President & CEO of a pharmaceutical multinational

We are accustomed to thinking that people think and act like us. Often this perception has been proven to be wrong, and has cost us dearly. And yet we continue to think this way.

If we were Mr. Smith, the first thing we would do on arriving at the office in the morning would be to ask our employees about the improvement in health we realized for our clients. We would be proud of the beneficial effects of our products. But we are not Mr. Smith.

As for Mr. Smith, he works for a multinational belonging to financiers. For them, only profits count. Mr. Smith graduated from business school with a sound background in productivity, finance, efficiency, and marketing. The bottom-line is the only thing that matters to him. He knows how to exploit his commodity: the public. His product: drugs. His evaluation criteria: the stock market. If the value of the shares grows, he will keep his job and receive a big bonus. If it dips, he will lose his job.

So what does Mr. Smith do when he arrives at the office in the morning. **He checks the stock market!**

Therefore it becomes clear that Mr. Smith:

1. Must **sell** as many drugs as possible. In order to achieve this, anything goes. Lies, fraud, concealing information, kickbacks, and so on. In the name of product excellence, he will resort to any manner of tactic to improve the firm's financial performance. He will put children, women, and men under medication, as well as the elderly. And he will vaccinate entire populations. All this with the connivance of the authorities. Both medical and governmental!

His marketing budget is 2 to 3 times that of research.

His principal salespeople are doctors. Mr. Smith trains them in medical schools where he controls the curriculum. Then he cultivates them through conventions and scientific publications that he finances. He provides them with information brochures for their waiting rooms. His staff monitors their billing charts.

He rewards them with research grants, gifts and perks such as trips. And entertains them lavishly.

His **principal buyers** are the public who he solicits directly via:

- magazines, "informative articles".
- newspapers, focusing on the launch of "new products" so that people will ask their doctors and pharmacists for them.
- foundations, which "inform" the public of the dangers of certain illnesses and diseases, of the need to prevent them, and the importance of helping those who have contracted the illness.
- public places like shopping centres and schools, where he presents information on sicknesses and their treatments.
- television, either directly in advertising his products, or indirectly in self-serving ads about the pharmaceutical industry's considerable research efforts.

Recently, when I was giving a course, I ate in the university cafeteria. *To my surprise , I saw a table, complete with video, pamphlets, and sellers busy informing the students of the dangers of hepatitis B, "AIDS WHICH CAN BE BEATEN", thanks to a vaccine which they were selling. Lies, manipulation, fear. Anything goes.*

Understand well, however, that selling shoes or selling vaccines/medications, it is selling!

How could these sellers be allowed or authorized to solicit the students? And with the blessing of the university authorities?

That's the establishment and its associates. You scratch my back, I'll... Let me sell... and I will give you your research project. All this dirty business under the hypocritical guise of information and education. And with our funds!

2. Makes sure that his products **only alleviate** problems but **do not cure** them, thus ensuring the financial performance of sickness.

3. Doesn't concern himself with the fact that his drugs **make people ill**. The fact is their harmful effects are extremely frequent and lead to the taking of still other drugs, which is simply good for business.

In January 1993, The Medical Information, a medical tabloid, reported that the Ministry of Health of Ontario had recently signed an agreement with the Burroughs Wellcome company to purchase zidovudine (Retrovir), which is used to treat people infected with the HIV virus. This three year agreement, engaged the Ministry to buy its stock of zidovudine from Burroughs Wellcome. In exchange, the pharmaceutical company undertook to invest $1.25 million annually into new social programs for those suffering from AIDS or who are HIV positive, as well as in research projects relating to the AIDS virus.

"Competition is a sin."

J.D. Rockefeller

4. Makes sure that his **medications be imposed**. He deals with bureaucrats who determine health expenditures.

5. Eliminates **competition**. From the producers of affordable generic counterparts to manufacturers of natural remedies. He also makes every effort to have the practice of alternative medicines banned. As he controls the medical and political authorities, this is not difficult.

In October 1994, on the NBC program Dateline, a doctor was asked about an alternative treatment for youngsters suffering from a form of epileptic seizures. The success of this treatment, a simple diet, has been shown (by Johns Hopkins, no less) to far outperform that of the drugs that were being generally prescribed. When asked why doctors did not promote or suggest this treatment to parents of children suffering from such seizures, he responded, rather sheepishly, that doctors did not because "there was no major drug company behind it".

The parents featured in the story had taken the initiative to read up on treatments for their child. All others had failed. They then followed through despite the advice of their doctor. Their child is reportedly doing much better. They have since set up a foundation to inform others of the availability of this treatment.

6. Seeks to **control** information, legislation, and the economic/financial decisions which impact upon his products. To achieve this, he sits on numerous boards of directors, belongs to secret societies, secret commissions, and leads a social active life geared to influence - peddling and lobbying.

7. Makes sure that **scientific research is profitable**. He ensures that his research costs are minimal, are supported and subsidized by public funds, are done in university facilities, and that they result in remedies that pay, for which he has the exclusive patent.

8. Makes sure that his products sell at the **highest price possible**. To achieve this, he patents them. The patent protects the monopoly of the product and, as a result, its monopolistic sales price. Mr. Smith patents all

that is patentable, and all that is not. He doesn't hesitate to have the U.N. and its bodies declare that some medicinal plants are a "world heritage". In this way, he can appropriate the exclusivity, patent them, and sell them at exorbitant prices, even to those who actually own them. Mr. Smith has even gone as far as creating from nothing, despite the protestations of the people concerned, the "RIGHTS OF INTELLECTUAL PROPERTY OVER BIOLOGICAL MATERIAL".

Two years ago, in Canada, there was a big controversy surrounding the extension of patents. The Canadian public learned what Free Trade was all about. It was going to cost them billions of dollars a year, because the pharmaceutical multinationals, under the Free Trade Agreement, were now demanding an extension of their patents from 17 to 20 years.

A patent is issued for an original medication that has been invented or discovered for the first time. In order to enable the pharmaceutical companies to recoup their research and marketing costs, they can apply for a patent. During this time, the company holding the patent can sell the product at any price it wishes, without any restrictions. Nobody else could compete. When the patent expires, others can then copy the product. Then prices invariably drop, generally speaking in the following proportions:

1 competitor, a drop of   20% from the original price
2 competitors, a drop of   40% from the original price
3 competitors, a drop of   80% from the original price

This is all to say that, even if the medication is sold only at 20% of the original price, it still is very profitable. Hardly surprising that the pharmaceutical multinationals' profits far outweigh that of most other manufacturers.

Beth Burrow reported in **Boycott Quarterly** : During an international conference on the Future of Intellectual Property Protection for Biotechnology, one of the panelists reported on the problems the industry was facing with **"environmentalists and those who would bring ethics and other irrational considerations to the table."** And nobody felt the need to contradict this declaration!

The corporate philosophy of the healthcare business

During a meeting which brought together 40 businessmen and women from different fields of specialization and different parts of Canada, one of the participants nonchalantly threw out the words "we, commodities" in referring to the people in general. No sooner were the words out of her mouth than half the people in the room were furious, outraged at being called commodities. The other half asked what was bugging them. This woman then proceeded to expound on the nature of corporate philosophy and found it quite normal to consider people as commodities.

In the corporate philosophy, the word "commodity" applies to all which can be exploited for maximum profit. That includes people, their health, their organs, their blood, their life, etc. Nothing is spared, there are no limits.

The traffic in organs is a very lucrative industry in some countries. In Mexico reportedly, they remove the eyes from perfectly healthy children to sell them in the US. With the tacit complicity of the authorities.

The traffic in blood is also a paying business. The authorities have not hesitated to authorize the use of contaminated blood to protect financial business interests. Even more, they still protect these business people and make us, the public, pay the costs of compensation. Costs that should be borne entirely by those responsible. Those who profited from the fraud.

The corporate philosophy of anything goes

This extends to schools, colleges, universities, where it is taught like a religion. We make heroes out of people who succeed by this philosophy. Success stories excite us all, and give us hope that we too can become like them. In this way, the establishment is able to continue its domination and exploitation for profit.

Even hospitals. Why are certain illnesses "welcome" in hospitals? Because they make money. Just as others are "refused". Because they do not. One only has to impose criteria of profitability on hospitals to determine which illnesses are treated or not. Who is treated or not.

Speaking of **profitability**, regardless of the field, it entails putting profits before the needs of clients. In medicine, this means sacrificing the health of many to line the pockets of a selected few. That is why government wants to control your health!

Some examples of "good business"

1. **Obesity**. As we know, obesity is more often than not the result of an under-lying emotional problem. But obesity pays. It generates vast sums of money for industry. Keeping people in a state of submission and making them feel abnormal and guilty is good business.

2. **Sterility**. This results in large part from pollution in the water, air, and foods we eat. Yet this pollution makes money for industry. Therefore, they don't touch it. Moreover, sterility opens the door to quite another lucrative business. That of *in vitro* fertilization.

3. **Breast cancer**. Cancer is the result of feelings of hopelessness and helplessness. Yet the authorities proclaim everywhere that one in 3...4...9 women will have breast cancer. It is persistently impressed upon our minds so that it will in fact happen. In addition, they push mammograms which create the fear of cancer and precipitate it. Which is good business.

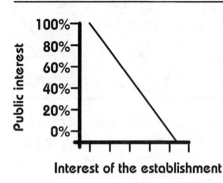

4. **Cholesterol**. This is not a sickness. But a number. A number that sells us pills which make us sick, which then sells more pills.

The higher the interest of the establishment, the lower our interest. The more the authorities recommend something, the greater our health is at risk.

5. **Depression.** It is a normal state in our evolution. It is a valley between two mountains. To have a depression is to descend one slope, to take stock, before climbing another. The last thing one needs in order to be able to climb out of it is drugs. They keep one in the valley, dependent on them. A bonanza of profits.

We live in an era that is seeing great transformations of our level of consciousness, which may be accompanied by bizarre physical and behavioral phenomena. Phenomena often inexplicable from a scientific viewpoint. Do not be worried. Live them. And above all, stop taking pills and drugs that are turning us into zombies.

Corporate philosophy versus common sense

- Corporate philosophy is learned in school. It is a way of thinking that is instilled in us by the authorities. It is external power.
- Common sense is not learned in school. On the contrary, it is suppressed. Common sense is our conscience which tells us whether we are in harmony with ourselves or not. It is our inner power which manifests itself. It is innate.

THE LONGER WE GO TO SCHOOL
THE LESS COMMON SENSE WE HAVE

CORPORATE PHILOSOPHY	COMMON SENSE
contrary to nature	natural
acquired	innate
rational	felt
instilled by the authorities	dictated by the conscience
external power	inner power
Instituted (DIS)ORDER	**Natural ORDER**

 To rediscover your common sense, forget about reason and listen to your heart, as you did when you were children. Have confidence in yourselves. You are divine.

The Trilogy of Lies

The lies of the authorities

For years, the authorities have been pulling the wool over our eyes. As we believe in the authorities, we unquestionably believe the truths they promulgate. It never occurs to us to doubt their sincerity. And yet...

Let us look closer at three of their lies.

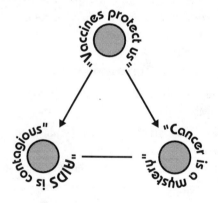

The trilogy of lies

PART ONE:
Vaccines protect us

*Do vaccines prevent illnesses...
or create them?*

We are taught by the authorities that vaccines protect us against eventual aggressive viruses and microbes and, therefore, prevent contagious illnesses and epidemics.

The big lie

This big lie has been perpetuated for 150 years despite the:

1. **INEFFECTIVENESS** of vaccines in protecting against illnesses:
   - vaccination may **provoke** the illness which it is supposed to prevent.
   - people who are vaccinated can **transmit** the illness, even if they are not ill themselves.
   - the vaccine can make the person more **susceptible** to the illness.

In 1905, the Philippines had a mortality rate of 10% due to smallpox. After a massive vaccination program, it reached epidemic proportions, killing 25% of the population, by now vaccinated. Despite this, the authorities stepped up the vaccinations. In 1918, the worst epidemic killed 54% of the people there, at a time when 95% of the population had been vaccinated. Manila, the capital, where everyone had been vaccinated or re-vaccinated, was the hardest hit with 65%. The Island of Mindanao, where the inhabitants had refused to be vaccinated, was the least hit. Only 11%. Despite this evidence, anti-smallpox vaccinations continued and, in 1966, the W.H.O. launched a world campaign which would last 10 years, only to be abandoned because it proved to be ineffective.

"The vaccinated child is a contaminated child"
Kalmar

2. **USELESSNESS** of certain vaccines, notably:
   - **Tuberculosis** and **tetanus** to which one is never immune. The fact that we have had tuberculosis does not prevent us from getting it again. On the contrary, a first case of tuberculosis, sometimes caused by the vaccine itself, renders one much more vulnerable to a second attack. And one that can be fatal.
   - **German measles** where 90% of women in a population are naturally protected and where the risk of contracting the sickness is limited to the first three months of pregnancy. Yet one vaccinates everybody.

- **Diphtheria** which is contracted by only 7% of children during the biggest epidemics. Yet again, everyone is vaccinated. Moreover, children and adults are vaccinated repeatedly, despite the fact that we are led to believe that one single vaccine received in childhood ensures immunity forever.

- **Influenza** and **hepatitis B** where the viruses rapidly become strongly resistant to antibodies of the vaccines. These two vaccines are therefore totally useless, in addition to being extremely dangerous.

"To vaccinate is to replace the natural immunity with an artificial immunity"

Simone Delarue

The best immunity is natural immunity. It is normally found in 80% to 90% of the population under the age of 15. Because the contamination of a person by an illness mobilizes all the body's defense systems, **natural immunization** goes hand in hand with being sick. Contamination from vaccines, on the other hand, short-circuits all the body's first line of defenses. **Artificial immunization** adds to the disorder. Hardly surprising that it requires to be repeated often. It is just as useless as the vaccines themselves!

3. Innumerable **COMPLICATIONS** of vaccines which go from minor problems (allergic, neurological) to death (sudden death of an infant) and which:

- are of short duration or permanent;
- immediately appear, later, much later;
- are short-lived or irreversible;
- are known and unknown.

Throughout my lectures and in discussions with people, I have made a list of the complications of vaccines that were communicated to me over the years. I relate these to you as such and have laid them out in the following table, according to when the complications appeared after the vaccination:

- rapidly (1 day to 1 month) SHORT TERM

- slowly (a few months to a few years) MEDIUM TERM

- much later (a few years to a few generations) LONG TERM

Complications in the short and medium term are known and documented. Complications in the long term are already evident in certain cases. But we do **not yet** have living proof for all. But do we want to wait until we see chicken wings appearing on our babies before we begin to ask questions?

A POT-POURRI OF COMPLICATIONS FROM VACCINATIONS

SHORT TERM	MID TERM	LONG TERM

The sickness itself or its atypical forms:
  - whooping cough
  - paralysis (polio-like)
Allergies
  - urticaria (giant)
  - eczema
  - exanthemes (rash)
  - asthma
  - discomfort and feeling faint
  - painful inflammations
  - local reactions
  - swollen ganglions
  - anaphylactic shock which can result in death
Fever
Renal attacks
Purpora
Edema (swelling)
Rheumatism
Gastro-intestinal problems
Unexpected infant death 1 to 3 weeks after vaccination
All acute illnesses of the nervous system:
  - serious to mild encephalitis
  - pan-encephalitis (measles vaccine)
  - meningitis
  - irreversible neurological attacks
  - Guillain-Barré
  - cerebral paralysis
  - major cerebral damage
"Vaccinal infarction" (30- and 40-year-olds)
Hepatitis B
Change or death of the fetus
	Neurological disorders
	1) **Autism**
	2) **Cerebral damage**
	  - convulsions
	  - hyperactive children
	  - incessant crying
	  - appetite problems (anorexia, bulimia)
	  - attack on cranial nerves (blindness/deafness/ dumb/dyslexia)
	  - hypotonia
	  - delayed development
	  - cerebral palsy
	3) **Mental problems**
	  - late mental development
	  - behavioral problems
	  - personality problems
	  - intellectual problems
	  - learning problems
	  - hyper-sexuality
	  - emotional instability
	  - juvenile delinquency
	  - sociopathic personality
	  - criminal behaviour
	Child leukemias
	Repetitive infections
	Numerous allergies
		DEFINITE EFFECTS
		1) Unbalancing of our body (individual ecology)
		2) Weakening of our immune system (natural defenses)
		3) Upsetting the interior of our cells: **permanent** alteration of chromosomes (DNA) (malformations)
		4) Introduction of foreign proteins **transmissible** to the genetic code of a species (new mutations)
		RESULTS
		  - multiple sclerosis
		  - leukemia
		  - cancer
		  - AIDS
		  - congenital malformations
		Sterility
		Chronic tiredness syndrome
		Epilepsy
		Parkinson's Disease
		Cardio-vascular illnesses
		Allergies +++
		Degenerative illnesses
		  - Alzheimer's
		  - Lupus
		  - Arthritis
		Re-appearance of old illnesses that are resistant to medications and drugs
		Appearance of new unknown illnesses
		  - Congenital malformations
		  - Hereditary genetic defects
		  - Mutations of the human species
		A threat of extinction for the human race

People who work with children, even once in a while, are reluctant to be vaccinated. I have a doctor friend who has always categorically refused to vaccinate against whooping cough. She prefers to be reprimanded by the authorities rather than having a death or an infirmity on her conscience. People who work with autistic children and/or those with behavioral or learning problems also know that there is nearly always a vaccination at the root of the problem. Recently, someone working with elderly people told me that her patients were sick for two or three months after they had received a vaccine against **influenza** and that many even died during this period.

4. Numerous **PROTESTATIONS** and **COMPLAINTS** continually repeated by specialists on the subject, conscientious doctors, and knowledgeable parents, or those who have children that are victims of vaccines. There are many reports of all kinds that are tucked away in filing cabinets. Out of sight, out of mind. The authorities have the information, but they hide it. It took them 45 years to reveal that 175,000 to 600,000 American soldiers were **contaminated** with hepatitis B when the virus was present in the vaccine against yellow fever!

> **Vaccination, Social Violence and Criminality - The Assault on the American Brain**
>
> Harris Coulter

5. **PARENT LEAGUES** and **ASSOCIATIONS**, such as
   - the *Dissatisfied Parents Together (DPT)* in the United States,
   - The *National League for the Freedom of Vaccinations* in France, which has been operational for 40 years and which has a well documented comprehensive library, has warned the authorities about the dangers of vaccinations and has claimed the right to **freedom of choice** for parents in matters of vaccination.

6. **LEGAL ACTIONS** are so numerous that they have threatened the very livelihood of certain manufacturers of vaccines. **Compensation funds** for victims of vaccines have been established by governments. One example is the *National Childhood Vaccination Compensation Law*, voted by Congress in December 1986, that authorizes the payment by government - with our dollars and not those of the responsible manufacturers - of damages to children seriously handicapped by a vaccination.

7. Catastrophic and staggering consequences of **EXTENSIVE NEUROLOGICAL DEFICIENCY**, which affects a great number of children, following on the heels of vaccinations. In the United States, 20% of youngsters suffer from developmental disabilities, as a result of encephalitis caused by vaccines. This, in turn, has had a profound **negative impact on the school system**, which is simply unable to accommodate so many children who can neither read nor write. It has also contributed to the marked increase in **social violence** and crimes committed by sociopathic personalities created by vaccines.

8. **FRIGHTENING AND UNFORESEEN EFFECTS**:
   - the **creation of new uncontrollable illnesses such as AIDS** and
   - the **permanent and hereditary changing of our genetic code**, the results of which we cannot even begin, or dare, to anticipate.

The following is a Government of Canada report entitled REPORT OF A VACCINE-ASSOCIATED ADVERSE EVENT. It is distributed to medical institutions.

Health and Welfare Canada / Santé de Bien être social Canada

In confidence to: Vaccine-Associated Adverse Events
Bureau of Communicable Disease
L.C.D.C., Tunney's Pasture
Ottawa, Ontario
K1A 0L2
(613) 957-1340

REPORT OF A VACCINE-ASSOCIATED ADVERSE EVENT

IDENTIFICATION

PATIENT	PROVINCE/TERRITORY	DATE OF BIRTH	Year	Month	Day	SEX ☐ Male ☐ Female	DATE OF VACCINE ADMINISTRATION	Year	Month	Day

VACCINES

VACCINE(S) GIVEN	NUMBER IN SERIES	ROUTE	DOSAGE	MANUFACTURER	LOT NUMBER	INTERVAL BETWEEN VACCINE ADMINISTRATION AND ONSET OF EVENT(S) (If more than one event reported below, record time to onset of the first event)
			☐ STANDARD OR SPEC. UNITS			_____ Minutes or
			☐ STANDARD OR SPEC. UNITS			_____ Hours or
			☐ STANDARD OR SPEC. UNITS			_____ Days

ADVERSE EVENT(S) (Report only events which cannot be attributed to co-existing conditions)

FEVER

☐ ≥40.5°C (105°F)

☐ 39.0-40.4°C (102.2-104.9°F)

☐ **TEMPERATURE NOT RECORDED** Believed to be very high AND presence of other systemic symptoms

LOCAL REACTION AT INJECTION SITE

☐ **INFECTIVE ABSCESS** Positive gram stain or culture

☐ **STERILE ABSCESS/NODULE/NECROSIS** No evidence of acute microbiological infection. Drainage, and/or nodule persisting more than one month and larger than 2.5 cm in diameter

☐ **SEVERE PAIN AND/OR SEVERE SWELLING** Lasting 4 days or more or requiring hospitalization; swelling past nearest joint as in arm past elbow

SYSTEMIC REACTION

☐ **ADENOPATHY** Severe or unusual enlargement or drainage of lymphatic nodes

☐ **ALLERGIC REACTION** Hives; wheezing; puffiness; generalized edema

☐ **RASHES** Severe – lasting 4 days or more or requiring hospitalization

☐ **ANAPHYLAXIS** Swelling of mouth/throat; difficulty breathing; shock; cardiovascular or respiratory collapse

☐ **HYPOTONIC – HYPORESPONSIVE EPISODE/EXCESSIVE SOMNOLENCE** Decrease/loss of muscle tone; loss of color/turning white or blue; decreased level/loss of consciousness; prolonged sleeping with difficulty arousing; cardiovascular or respiratory arrest

☐ **ARTHRALGIA/ARTHRITIS** Lasting over 24 hours

☐ **SEVERE VOMITING AND/OR DIARRHEA** Must interfere with daily routine

NEUROLOGIC SYMPTOMS/DIAGNOSIS

☐ **SCREAMING EPISODE/PERSISTENT CRYING** Unconsolable for 3 hours or more or quality of cry definitely abnormal for child and not previously heard by parents

☐ **CONVULSION/SEIZURE** Muscle contractions and decreased level of consciousness. May or may not be associated with fever

☐* **ENCEPHALOPATHY** Focal and diffuse neurologic signs; Increased intracranial pressure and/or changes lasting at least 6 hours in level of consciousness, with/without convulsions

☐* **MENINGITIS AND/OR ENCEPHALITIS**

☐* **ANAESTHESIA/PARAESTHESIA** Lasting over 24 hours

☐* **PARALYSIS**

☐* **GUILLAIN-BARRÉ SYNDROME** Progressive weakness of more than one limb and generalized hypo/areflexia

☐* **SUBACUTE SCLEROSING PANENCEPHALITIS (SSPE)**

MISCELLANEOUS

☐ **PAROTITIS** Swelling with pain and/or tenderness of parotid gland(s)

☐ **ORCHITIS** Swelling with pain and/or tenderness of testicle(s)

☐* **THROMBOCYTOPENIA**

☐ **OTHER SEVERE OR UNUSUAL EVENTS** (Please describe)

_____

_____

_____

*MUST BE DIAGNOSED BY A PHYSICIAN (Please give details)

OUTCOME OF EVENT(S) AT TIME OF REPORT	☐ Patient Recovered	PLEASE FORWARD ANY FOLLOW UP INFORMATION ☐ Patient recovered with residual effects	☐ Pending	☐ Unknown	☐ Fatal

HOSPITALIZED BECAUSE OF EVENT(S)	☐ NO	☐ YES	▶ Date Admitted	Year	Month	Day	Date Discharged	Year	Month	Day

REPORTER'S NAME

TELEPHONE NUMBER Area Code

COMMENTS

ADDRESS (No., Street, etc.)

City   Province   Postal Code

SIGNATURE   DATE Year Month Day

HPB 5127 (12 88)

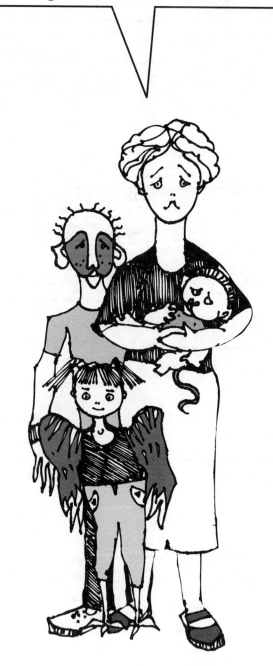

New types of viruses are creating themselves, transforming themselves, multiplying, and passing themselves on from one generation to another. They do so through sperm or the egg, placenta, or a mother's milk. Yet, several vaccines are made with viruses from cells of animals that are themselves contaminated with all sorts of viruses. And that is why we had some very unpleasant surprises:

- In 1960, cultures from the renal cells of rhesus monkies used in the manufacture of anti-polio vaccine were discovered to be infested with simian virus 40 (SV 40). As a result, millions of children were contaminated with this virus before it was detected. Today, however, we know that SV 40 causes a deficiency in the immune system, congenital anomalies, forms of leukemia (particularly in children aged two to four), as well as malignant illnesses.

- In 1973, researchers proved that the incidence of brain tumors was 13 times higher among children born of mothers who had been vaccinated against poliomyelitis during their pregnancy.

- In 1980, researchers found presence of SV 40 in human brain tumors. They seemed to be present in 25% of cases.

- In 1987, it was confirmed that HTLV4 came from green African monkeys. Yet the virus of human leukemia is HTLV1 and the virus of human AIDS is HTLV3. It is the same for the fowl leukosis virus which contaminated the yellow fever and measles vaccines until 1962. And then we ask WHY THERE IS AN AIDS EPIDEMIC?

The ransom of vaccinations
F. and S. Delarue

DESPITE ALL THAT, the authorities not only continue vaccinating our children from the cradle to the classroom, but they extend the practice to adults. Moreover, for the past 20 years, they have done so throughout the entire world.

Did you know that 45% of Unicef funds goes to vaccinating people in the Third World, compared to only 17% for clean water and sanitation? This despite the fact that, according to this same agency, one person in five in the world is not always served by water and a reliable sanitation system. Youngsters in the Third World need clean drinking water and food in their stomachs, not aggressive agents, which make them die like flies. Massive vaccinations in African countries have decimated these populations as a result of their immediate effects. And now as a result of AIDS. And yet we continue to vaccinate them regardless.

Better still, the world authorities have launched the Expanded Program on Immunization, the objective of which is to vaccinate all the children in the world against six illnesses that are most common among youngsters. Poliomyelitis, diphtheria, tetanus, measles, whooping cough, and tuberculosis.

Let us all realize that what the authorities are telling us is more often than not far different from the reality.

| Vaccination prevents epidemics | The real epidemic is vaccination |

The world authorities

The world government is the United Nations Organization, the U.N. Its Ministry of Health is the World Health Organization, W.H.O. The world government is in the process of imposing itself everywhere on the globe,

THE NEW WORLD ORDER

An all-powerful global authority, the government of governments, said to **ensure peace in the world**. With the purest of intentions, the U.N., through its Ministry of Health, W.H.O., has succeeded in achieving the following:

- In 1974, W.H.O. launched a massive program to promote "Health for all in the year 2000". This program was the result of a long battle led by people living in the Third World who finally convinced the organization that they had their own special needs and that they wanted to be part of the decision-making process.

It was also the time of the canonisation of W.H.O. - Saint W.H.O. - consecrated as the world authority in health matters. As a result, it would now assume responsibility for directing the focus and orientation of health in the world, overshadowing all national governments.

- In 1978, the Member States of W.H.O. met at Alma Ata to define a common policy of primary healthcare in which all their respective country's populations would be democratically involved. So that they themselves would be able to confront their own health problems. Yet we have seen earlier in this book, the Declaration of Alma Ata followed from the globalization of the recommendations of the Flexner Report. A report that imposed "scientific" medicine (medicine of sickness) as the only valid one, and eliminated all other medical practices. Let us not forget that this Report was financed by the Carnegie Foundation, and its application by the Rockefeller Foundation. The sponsors of the Alma Ata Conference included: the Rockefeller Foundation, the World Bank, and Unicef. Financiers magnanimously spending their money for the health of the world!

- In 1983, in order to achieve its praiseworthy objective of "health for all in the year 2000", Saint W.H.O. launched its Expanded Program on Immunization. A committee to oversee the vaccination of the children of the world against the six illnesses is established, comprising:

- Robert McNamara, former president of the World Bank, the official bank of the world government, the U.N.

- Jonas Salk, director of the Salk Institute, manufacturer of vaccines and biological reagents, most notably for the American army. The Salk Institute has a department which works under contract with the Pentagon. (In 1988, The Wall Street Journal reported that the Institute had concluded a $32 million deal with the Army to produce vaccines and biological reagents.)

- Léopold Sedar Senghor, former president of Senegal.

- Van den Hoven, president of Unilever, the huge multinational with interests in the Third World, whose speciality is to impose there the peanut mono-culture. Unilever is the most important manufacturer of margarine, oil, and soap in the world.

Saint W.H.O., financiers, industrialists, and militarists come together to save the children of the world. How touching!

- In 1984, in order to realize the pious wishes of Saint W.H.O., five respectable institutions combined forces and founded the Intervention Force for the Survival of Children, so as to continue and enlarge the vaccination program on a global scale: Saint W.H.O., Unicef, the World Bank, the U.N. Development Program and the Rockefeller Foundation. Unicef is encouraged in its noble venture by the Mérieux Foundation, which has 30% of the world's vaccine manufacturing market, and the Pasteur Institute. What generosity!

- In 1989, in order to impose immunization programs on children as fore-seen by the Expanded Program on Immunization, as well as beat the resis-tance and opposition put up by obstinate adults, Saint W.H.O. went in search of a restraining tool. Always for the good of the children, of course. It had the U.N. adopt the Convention of Rights of the Child to improve the lot of children in the world. This convention unilaterally and arbitrarily imposed fundamental changes in the structure of our society and our fami-ly. Without any discussion, representation or consultation with citizens whatsoever!

In practice, this Convention:

a) establishes the concept of **citizenship** of the child.

b) replaces the right of authority of the parents with a **duty to obey** the administrative authorities.

c) enables the authorities to separate the child from neglectful parents.

d) recognizes the child has freedom of choice, thought, expression, to practice his, or her religion or convictions, association, and peaceful gatherings, **the only restrictions** being those which are prescribed by law, or which relate to **health**.

e) prescribes that all countries do all in their power to ensure the integral realization of the right of the child to enjoy a better state of health and take the appropriate measures to develop **preventive healthcare**, including vaccination.

The Convention of Rights of the Child allows the authorities to impose by force, against the wishes of the parents:

- blood transfusions to those who may oppose them.
- vaccines to those who oppose them.
- scientific medicine to those who may prefer alternative medicines.
- severe medical treatments to those who refuse them, such as AZT for AIDS.

Let us not lose sight of the fact that it is not

✔ children, nor parents,

✔ nor our children,

✔ nor we, the patients,

✔ nor our doctors,

✔ nor the authorities of our country,

but rather the **world financiers** who control our health, hidden behind the respected Saint W.H.O.

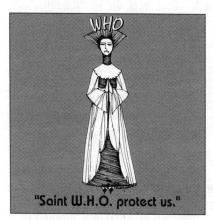

"Saint W.H.O. protect us."

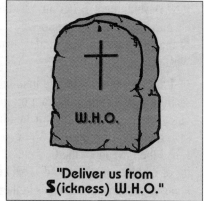

"Deliver us from **S**(ickness) W.H.O."

Why this lethal relentlessness?

What is the objective of the world authorities in destroying people's health, **both in industrialized countries and in the Third World**? It is always diffi-cult to presume the intentions of others, particularly when one is not close to them. And this is true in this instance. But there are certainly advantages for someone, somewhere, to so doggedly keep-up the campaign for vaccinations, by any and all means possible. They must profit someone, somewhere. One thing is certain. It is not to our advantage. In order to determine what these advantages are, and for whom, let us stop and look at the CONSEQUENCES of these massive vaccination programs and draw our own conclusions.

1. Vaccination is expensive and represents a cost of **one billion dollars annually**. It therefore benefits the industry, most notably, the multinational manufacturers. One sells the vaccines. The other then provides the arsenal of medications to respond to the numerous complications that follow. Their profits increase while our expenses go through the roof. To the point where we have simply had it up to here and are ready to accept the unacceptable, such as socialized medicine in the United States, for example.

2. Vaccination stimulates the immune system, the body's defense mechanism. Repeated, vaccination exhausts the immune system. It gives a false sense of security and, in doing so, it opens the door wide to all kinds of illnesses. Notably, to those related to AIDS, which can only develop on ripe ground, where the immune system has been disturbed. It causes AIDS to explode. It ensures that the illness flourishes perpetually.

3. Vaccination leads to social violence and crime. What better way to **destabilize** a country than to **disarm** its inhabitants, and reinforce police and military control? The authorities subtly create situations of panic and fear among the population which, in turn, necessitate the reinforcement of "protection measures", including forbidding citizens from owning weapons. The authorities then come across as saviors and strengthen their control. It is certain that, in order to impose a single world army, one must first disarm the citizens of every country. One must therefore create violence, if they are to achieve this disarmament, particularly in the United States where the right to bear arms is guaranteed by the Constitution.

4. Vaccination encourages medical **dependence** and reinforces belief in the inefficiency of the body. It creates people who need permanent assistance. It replaces the confidence one has in oneself with a blind confidence in others, outside ourselves. It leads to loss of personal dignity, in addition to making us financially dependent. It draws us into the vicious circle of sickness (fear - poverty - submission) and, in this way, ensures the **submission of the herd** so as to better dominate and exploit it. And then lead them to the abattoir. To slaughter.

   Vaccination also encourages the moral and financial dependence of Third World countries. It perpetuates the social and economic control of Western countries over them.

5. Vaccination camouflages the **real socio-political problems** of poverty of some due to exploitation by others, and results in techno-scientific pseudo-solutions that are so complicated and sophisticated that patients cannot understand them. In addition, vaccination diverts funds which should be used to help improve living conditions, and channels them into the banks of the multinationals. It widens the gap between the dominant rich and the exploited poor.

   complexity
   =
   control

6. Vaccination **decimates populations**. Drastically in Third World countries. Chronically in industrialized countries. In this regard, the former President of the World Bank, former Secretary of State in the United States, who ordered massive bombing of Vietnam, and member of the Expanded Program on Immunization, Robert McNamara, made some very interesting remarks. As reported by a French publication, *"J'ai tout compris"*, he was quoted as stating:

   "One must take draconian measures of demographic reduction against the will of the populations. Reducing the birth rate has proved to be impossible or insufficient. One must therefore increase the mortality rate. How? By natural means. Famine and sickness." (Translation)

7. Vaccination enables the selection of populations to be decimated. It facilitates **targeted genocide**. It permits one to kill people of a certain race, a certain group, a certain country. And to leave others untouched. In the name of health and well-being, of course.

   Take Africa, for example. We have witnessed the almost total disappearance of certain groups. Some 50% dead, estimate the most optimistic. Some 70% dead, according to the less optimistic. As if by chance, many were in the same region, such as Zaire, Uganda, the extreme south of the Sudan. In 1967, at

Marburg in Germany, seven researchers, working with green African monkeys, died of an unknown hemorrhagic fever. In 1969, also by chance, the same sickness killed one thousand people in Uganda. In 1976, a new unknown hemorrhagic fever killed in the south of Sudan. Then in Zaire.

It is noteworthy that since1968, virologists (virus specialists) have installed their sophisticated equipment in certain hospitals in Zaire.

At a CIA hearing, Dr. Gotlieb, a cancerologist, admitted having dispersed, in 1960, a large quantity of viruses in the Congo River (in Zaire) to pollute it and contaminate all the people who used the river as their source of water. Dr. Gotlieb was named to head up the *National Cancer Institute!*

A couple of years ago, Reuters reported: "An illness similar to AIDS has killed 60,000 in the south of Sudan. They call the illness, the killer. Families, whole villages, have disappeared. This illness, the Kala-azar, takes the form of a fever and loss of weight. The symptoms are the same as those of AIDS. The immune system is deficient and one dies of other infections."

> "Is paranoia a form of awareness?"
>
> Kerry Thornley

It is obvious that Africa, particularly those countries in the center and to the south, contain fabulous resources that have always incited westerners to crush their inhabitants to take over their riches. And beware anyone who stands in their way. The colonies have disappeared. But not colonialism.

8. Vaccination serves as a form of **experimentation**, to test new products on a great sampling of a population. Under the guise of health and the well-being of the population, people are vaccinated against a pseudo-epidemic with products that one wants to study. The **vaccine of hepatitis B** seems to be the choice of authorities to accomplish this goal. Yet, this vaccine is manufactured by a process of genetic manipulation. And it is much more dangerous than the traditional vaccine because it inoculates into the body cells that are foreign to its genetic code. Moreover, this vaccine is produced from virus cultivated on the ovaries of Chinese hamsters. One can only imagine what future generations will look like! But there is more. It is also reported to cause cancer of the liver. Despite all that, it enjoys great popularity among the authorities, who impose it first on all those who work in the health field, and then on the rest of the population.

> experimentation = extermination of bothersome minorities

• In 1986, the medical authorities administered the vaccine against **hepatitis B** to Native Indian children in Alaska, without any explanation or the consent of their parents. Many children fell ill. And several died. It seems there was a virus called *RSV (Rous Sarcoma Virus)* in the vaccine.

American Indian tribes have been subjected to many vaccinations. Let us be aware that they are **difficult to beat into submission**, and they own vast tracts of land which the authorities would like to have for their own benefit.

Recently, when I met a group of Native women to chat about health with them, the subject of vaccinations cropped up. I was giving them some information on the topic when, suddenly, the group's nurse confided in me that the federal government had given her complete freedom in the management of their health, but on one strict condition. That every vaccination had to be scrupulously applied to all. The silence was deafening. We all understood.

- In 1988, the Ambassador of Senegal gave a radio interview reporting on the ravages of AIDS in his country where entire villages were being decimated. A few years earlier, scientific and medical teams had come to vaccinate their inhabitants against **hepatitis B**.

- In 1978, a new vaccine was tested on homosexuals in New York. And in 1980, on those in San Francisco, Los Angeles, Denver, Chicago, and St-Louis. Officially, this "new vaccine" was against **hepatitis B** and, as we now know, it caused many of them to die from AIDS. It sounded the "official" beginning of the AIDS epidemic in 1981.

The vaccination program of homosexuals against **hepatitis B** was led by Saint W.H.O. and the *National Institute of Health* . There are reports of collaboration between these two organizations in 1970 to study the consequences of certain viruses and bacteria introduced to children during vaccination campaigns. In 1972, they transformed this study to focus on the viruses which provoked a drop in the immune mechanism.

Wolf Szmuness directed the anti-**hepatitis B** experiments undertaken in New York. He had very close links with the *Blood Centre* where he had his laboratory, the *National Institute of Health*, the *National Cancer Institute*, the *F.D.A.*, the W.H.O., and the Schools of Public Health of Cornell, Yale, and Harvard.

In 1994 a vast vaccination campaign against **hepatitis B** was undertaken in Canada. It is both useless, dangerous and costly. And what for? Is there a hidden agenda? I note that the Province of Quebec is a particular target, over the course of three years.

- 1992: vaccination against meningitis
- 1993: re-vaccination against meningitis
- 1994: vaccination against **hepatitis B**.

I was there in 1993. It troubled me to see that it was aimed at a whole generation (1 to 20 years), in only one province. Since when do viruses respect borders, and specially provincial ones at that? The facts are:

- There was no epidemic, nor risk of one. Epidemiologists confirmed it.
- Not one but three different vaccines were administered, each in a desinated area.
- Certain nurses were selected and trained to administer a special vaccine.
- All children were entered into a computerized data bank.
- The pressure to vaccinate the children was enormous. Schools were turned into clinics. Those who did not want to be vaccinated were pointed out and treated as social outcasts.
- Nurses chased down parents at home who did not want their pre-school children vaccinated.

I had a direct account of one of these kids. The mother did not want her child vaccinated. The nurse who came to the house made her believe that it was compulsory. The mother gave in... The child is now handicapped: physically and mentally (paralyzed, spastic).

- The vaccination cost $30 million.

Why was there such a murderous will. Like Native peoples, the people of Quebec are also a "bother". They believe in their cultural identity and in sovereignty. What is more, Quebec with its Native territories, encompasses huge reservoirs of water which many a multinational have their eyes on. As an acquaintance of mine who sits on the California water management board said, "Water today is gold." Could one think of a more appropriate biological weapon to possibly remove any impediments to accessing that resource?

9. Vaccinations permit **epidemiological studies** of populations to collect data on the resistance of different ethnic groups to different illnesses. It permits one to study the reactions of the immune systems of large numbers of the population to an antigen (virus, microbe) injected by vaccination. Should it be within the framework of the fight against an existing illness, or one that has been provoked.

- In 1987, certain American laboratories and the Department of Biotechnology of India signed an agreement authorizing the testing of genetically manufactured vaccines on the people of India. This agreement was met with fierce opposition because it gave access to epidemiological and immunity profiles of a population. This data is extremely important from a military standpoint. It is even more valuable because India has never experienced yellow fever. And, at time of writing this book, it had known only a handful case of AIDS. Over and above all that, the private American laboratories proposed to test products on the Indian population for which they had no right to test in the United States! And the Indian authorities acquiesced!

10. Vaccination is a **biological weapon** at the service of **biological warfare**. It permits the targeting of people of a certain race, and leaves the others who are close by more or less untouched. It makes it possible to intervene in the hereditary lineage of anyone selected. A new speciality is born. **Genetic engineering**. It is flourishing, enjoys much prestige, and is receiving substantial research funds. The challenge is staggering. To find a vaccine which gives an illness against which we already have the vaccine! In this way, we would be able to send in troops who have already been vaccinated against the killer vaccine, which they would then spread among the enemy. **It is absolutely crazy and insane!**

Meanwhile, **industrial theft** is in full swing. Captain and biologist of the *US Navy* at Fort Detrick, Neil Levitt, reported the disappearance of 2.35 liters of an experimental vaccine. A dose sufficient to contaminate the entire world. Fort Detrick is a research laboratory which manufactures vaccines. It is located quite close to Washington, in Maryland, and it is attached to the *National Cancer Institute* at Bethesda, a suburb of the capital.

It is hardly astonishing that, in every major vaccination campaign, one finds the same tangled web. Government, the military, Saint W.H.O., financiers, researchers, laboratories, universities, the CIA, and the World Bank.

Let us not lose sight of the fact that:

In the name of the defense of our countries, we manufacture the most murderous of weapons. War, whether it be biological or not, is war. And weapons kill. Biological warfare is a giant business, largely financed **BY OUR FUNDS**, through the medium of the military, research, and our donations. It is also financed, and without our knowledge, **BY OUR LIVES**. Those of our children and of millions of innocents who have been sacrificed. It is we, those who live in the Western world, who are responsible for all the illnesses and acts of genocide in the world. By our acceptance of vaccinations, both at home and abroad.

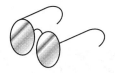

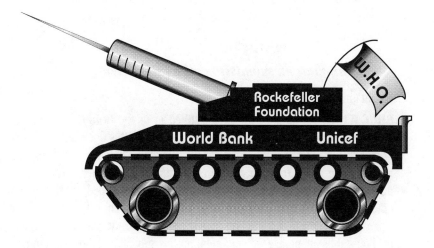

Social marketing

MARKETING is a relatively recent "science" that encompasses several disciplines, such as information, advertising, education, influence, lobbying, press releases, messages, jingles, gadgets, and the like. It may be written, oral, silent, subliminal. It may be open, subtle, or hidden. It is the science of manipulation. It is taught at university. One hands out diplomas. One creates specialists. Regardless of the nature of the actual product, the goal is to create a demand, or a need, on the part of the "consumer". To cause people to purchase products that they might not normally buy. Because they don't really want them or because they don't really need them.

SOCIAL MARKETING, also called social engineering, is identical to conventional marketing except for the product it promotes. **It sells ideas**, that is, it gets people to accept the ideas of someone else and to make them their own. Specially ideas that run contrary to their own or to their common sense. The goal of social marketing is the **submission** of the conscience, to put the conscience to sleep in order to lead us down a path. With our full consent. It replaces conscience. And with it, undermines our power to choose. It is what Beauvais and Joule call "submission freely consented to". They add: "In the final analysis, it allows one to think, decide, and conduct oneself in total freedom. But differently from how one would do so spontaneously".

MEDICAL SOCIAL MARKETING is the science of social marketing applied to the field of health. It consists of SELLING SICKNESS TO PEOPLE WHO WANT HEALTH.

SOCIAL MARKETING OF VACCINATION is to sell the idea of the necessity of vaccination to people who do not need, or want it. The target goal is to submit 95% of the population to all vaccinations that the authorities decide they should have. This involves three stages, which intensify according to the degree of resistance to the submission.

a) manipulation

b) organization

c) repression

Ist stage, manipulation: submission with full consent

It contaminates all fields:

- **EDUCATION.** The authorities have instilled in us the **belief** that vaccinations are effective and harmless. Whoever questions this doctrine, be they a doctor or non-doctor, is a heretic. Yet we have come to learn that the reality is something else altogether. There is more. The authorities scrupulously uphold another **myth**. Namely, that vaccinations have wiped out the major epidemics. Yet these major epidemics had almost entirely disappeared when the vaccines first came on the market. Books on vaccines, not written by the establishment, are very eloquent on this subject and they substantiate this fact as far as every one of the former major illnesses is concerned.

  It is improvement in living conditions, and notably that of hygiene, that has caused the progressive disappearance of illnesses that once were the scourge of the planet. Ivan Illich also confirms this in his respected book, **Medical Nemisis**. This brainwashing is called **"sanitary education"** or **"public hygiene"**. Everyone working in the health field receives this deceitful training regarding vaccination. They pass it on, without questioning it. And in doing so, they transform vaccination into an aggression which becomes normal. Just like violence and war on television.

- **VOCABULARY.** The authorities put words in our mouth which shape our ideas and the way we behave. For example, winter is referred to as **"the season of the common cold"**. From this stems the concept of a cold epidemic and the need for vaccination against it. And we're hooked! But social marketing goes further. It makes us believe that the elderly are more vulnerable to illnesses, including colds in winter, and therefore of the necessity to **vaccinate them all**. And, to provide them with even greater protection, everyone involved in treating them must also be vaccinated! This is what one calls "gerontocide".

The refrigerator has done more for health than open-heart surgery

"It is easier for a man to split an atom than to break a preconception"
A. Einstein

One of the initiators of the vaccine against the common cold frequently repeated to friends: "If you want to inherit quickly, vaccinate your grandmother against a cold!"

- **EMOTIONS.** Not just any. But fear. The very concept of vaccination rests on the **FEAR-PROTECTION TANDEM**. They make us afraid so that we will run after a savior to protect us. Are we so helpless and ill-equipped that we have need of protection? Manipulation makes us believe that we do. We allow ourselves to be taken care of by our protectors. Just like with the Mafia. But protection does not come cheaply! So as to be even more effective, social marketing plays upon another emotion. One that is even more perverse. **Guilt**. "If I do not vaccinate my child and he becomes ill, I would never forgive myself as long as I live. And if he suddenly dies in his crib, or gets leukemia at three years old, or multiple sclerosis when he is older, because we did not have him vaccinated, what will we give as a reason?" Let us realize that there is no end to it. Nor does it make sense. Moreover, who are we to take upon ourselves responsibility for the death of others?

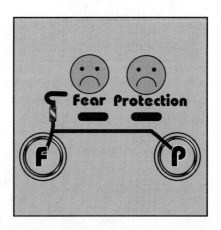

- **INFLUENCE**. One must do like the others. If everyone else does it, then it must be good. But have we forgotten the Pied Piper of Hamlin? That is submission. And that is what it leads to. We follow fashion fads in clothing, foods, music. And vaccinations. Above all, don't question. The authorities know better than us. And they tell us that all is well. Who are we to dare think any differently? One calls that **social pressure**. It is orchestrated by the *establishment & associates:* financial, political, industrial, medical, insurance, religious, artistic, and academic. It is disseminated by social marketing.

- **MORALITY**. The authorities speak of the "right to health for all". Who could put it better? Yet whoever speaks of a right speaks of a duty. And from here stems the concept of a **"social duty"** to be vaccinated. To refuse to do so would be to refuse health for all. What a lack of ethics and social conscience! And being a good citizen, we fulfill our duties and get vaccinated. And social marketing has met its goal.

- **INFORMATION.** Medical or non-medical, information is in the hands of the establishment to serve its own ends. It is the tool of broadcasting social marketing. Many journalists transmit **information which comes to them from the authorities** and simply reproduce it faithfully, without doubting it for one minute. Particularly when it comes to the highly protected subject of vaccination, they hesitate to stray from the beaten path and ask questions. If they ask too many, their text is cut. Then their job. Be that as it may, some have questioned. For example, in 1979, the CBS television program

"60 Minutes" presented an inquiry on the massive vaccination campaign against **swine fever** in the United States in 1976. This vaccine created so many complications, particularly neurological, resulting in death or paralysis, that the manufacturers were inundated with massive legal actions and the vaccine was suspended. This broadcast was the showcase of social marketing in all its glory. All the elements are there. I strongly recommend that you get a copy of the video or a transcript to see how one organizes a massive vaccination campaign.

2nd stage, organization: submission with LESS consent

This ensures the effectiveness of the manipulation. It comprises a system of **control by computer index** of the population and of doctors. All are tabulated on a computer, which ensures that they can be tracked down. In this way, the authorities ensure that every citizen regularly receives his or her vaccines and that every doctor is involved. Lists are drawn up. Indexes tabulated. Vaccination report cards issued. Nobody can escape. Those who are negligent are immediately called to order and are brought in line. It is systematic regimentation. *BIG BROTHER* is watching your health!

3rd stage, repression: submission with NO consent

It punishes insubordination. In order to ensure obedience, the authorities make laws. Vaccines became obligatory at the very beginning of the century. They still are in many countries. When people become aware of the reality of vaccinations, the seeds of rebellion are sown. Whenever resistance becomes too strong, the World Health Organization quietly passes new laws, such as the Convention of Rights of the Child.

- Those who disobey are forbidden access to nurseries, schools, universities, certain hospitals or clinics. They cannot travel abroad. They are forbidden from practicing certain professions. They are continually harassed by the medical, administrative, and school authorities. They are the black sheep in the beautiful program of "health for all".
- The very rebellious are hit with fines, lose their right to practice medicine, are put in prison, or are vaccinated by force.

Let us not lose sight of the fact that:

This hierarchal network is directed on a **national** scale by each country's "ministry of health", Donna Governmenta, herself under the directive of the **world** "ministry of health", Saint W.H.O.

In conclusion

The words of American doctor, Edward Kasse, who addressed the Convention of Vienna on Infectious Diseases in 1983, in his role as president of the Convention, speak for themselves:

"The goal of epidemiologists should not be the irradication of infectious diseases thanks to the massive use of vaccines and antibiotics, but rather the control and improvement of the quality of life. One must admit that there exists a certain number of cases of tuberculosis, polio or malaria and enter into a natural, ecological dynamic in making more effective the possibilities of our body's defenses, thanks to a health policy that is not contaminated by the interests of pharmaceutical multinationals."

In the final analysis, we find ourselves once again facing the following dilemma. Obey the authorities or listen to our conscience. Give our power to others or exercise it ourselves. Blame our governments or assume our own responsibilities. **It is a question of conscience**. To this effect, there do exist "clauses of conscience" which are recognized in certain American States for one to refuse vaccination. In France, young people recruited into the army have the same legal right. In Canada, vaccination is a matter of choice, but we are led to believe that it is obligatory. The right to health is a legitimate, innate right of every human being. No law can grant us that which we already have. And even less, take it away from us. To obey the laws is to submit to **legality**, exterior power. Listening to one's conscience is to respect its **legitimacy**. Its inner power of divine essence. Between legality and legitimacy, WE HAVE THE POWER TO CHOOSE!

Banco Mondialo

Saint-WHO

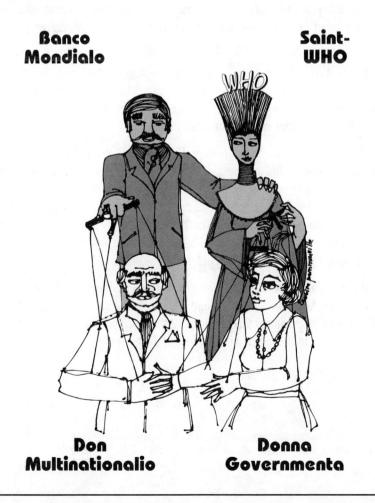

Don Multinationalio

Donna Governmenta

The trilogy of lies

PART TWO:
AIDS is contagious

AIDS is caused only by the HIV virus
... or by the use of drugs, medications, vaccines?

What is AIDS?

Acquired
Immuno-
Deficiency
Syndrome

ACQUIRED, that is to say obtained, contrary to the natural, innate, heredi-tary. THEREFORE, the weakening of our defense system is acquired during the course of our life. WHERE, WHEN, HOW? That is the question. And the enigma!

IMMUNO for immunity. This is the natural or acquired resistance of a living organism to an infectious agent (microbe, virus) or to a toxic agent (venom, toxins).

DEFICIENCY, that is to say organic or physical insufficiency. THEREFORE, different illnesses have in common an immuno-deficiency. Namely, an insuffi-ciency on the part of the body to resist, a weakness of the body's defense system. From where it becomes easy to contract illnesses.

SYNDROME comes from Greek and means reunion. It is a clearly defined combination of signs and symptoms which can be seen in many different illness-es and which does not allow one in and of itself to determine the cause and the nature of the illness. Take, for example, the cold syndrome. The signs and symp-toms are well known. Discomfort, fever, cramps, tiredness, a runny nose, watery eyes. We know that this involves a cold. But we cannot determine what kind of cold we have, nor the cause of the cold. It is the same for AIDS.

It is a combination of signs and symptoms. Tiredness, weakness, loss of appetite, fever, infections, loss of weight. The same that we find in many illness-es. It is not only one illness that can present these symptoms, but many different illnesses. It remains to determine the cause of these illnesses.

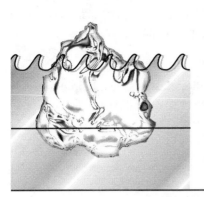

Symptoms:	-Tiredness -Fever -Infections -Anorexia
AIDS	
Causes of immuno-deficiency:	-Submission -Fear -Poverty -Drugs

We note that with the one definition of the letters A-I-D-S and based on our common sense, we can arrive at an understandable definition of AIDS:

- AIDS IS A COMBINATION OF **SYMPTOMS** (the tip of the iceberg).

- PRESENT IN DIFFERENT ILLNESSES (the body of the iceberg)

WHICH HAVE IN COMMON A **WEAKNESS OF THE DEFENSE SYSTEM.**

- THE CAUSE OF THIS WEAKNESS IS **ACQUIRED**

SOMEWHERE IN THE COURSE OF OUR LIFE (the base of the iceberg).

Causes of AIDS

The entire question is there. Because a good diagnosis leads to a good treatment. If the illnesses of AIDS have an immunitary weakness in common, it is logical to direct our efforts towards the causes in order to cure the illness. And, particularly, to prevent it. The most frequent **CAUSES OF IMMUNITARY WEAKNESS** among people who are sick with one of the illnesses of AIDS are:

1. Indiscriminate use of **illegal drugs**. It seems to be the most devastating. One must not only stop the use of contaminated syringes, but the use of drugs itself.

   To prevent is to avoid having to cure

2. **Medications:** antibiotics, anti-inflammatories, chemotherapy, transfusions, blood derivatives. "We are an immune-depressed society", states Dr. McKenna. In the United States, for example, every year sees $30 billion in prescribed medications and $50 billion in non-prescribed medications (over the counter).

3. **Vaccines**. We know that vaccines depress the immune system. Children receive some 20 vaccines before starting school. Then people of all ages are submitted to annual vaccinations and, occasionally, to mass vaccinations.

4. **Pollution** of the air, water, foodstuffs. Countless industrial chemical products pollute the water that we drink and the air which we breathe. Moreover, our foodstuffs are filled with radioactivity, electromagnetic waves, pesticides and chemical fertilizers. And that is not even including the vaccines and hormones that are present in the meat we eat.

5. **Malnutrition**. Whether it be by scarcity, dieting, excess, or alcoholism. It goes hand in hand with infectious illnesses. It is particularly present in Third World countries and among pregnant women.

6. Recurring **infections** of all kinds, acute or chronic.

7. Factors which affect a person's soul. **Hopelessness** and **helplessness**. A feeling that one's life lacks any purpose or sense of direction. Submission to fatal prognosis.

8. A libertine or unbalanced **lifestyle**.

9. **Lack of love** and caring support.

10. **Fear** which imprisons us. It is our worst enemy.

At the Convention of Copenhagen on AIDS, in May 1992, "surviving" patients of AIDS all agreed. To live, one must correct the causes of the immuno-deficiency. And first and foremost, one must free oneself from fear. It kills us. Other solutions proposed by scientific medicine are ineffective, particularly AZT. None of their friends who had taken AZT, a strong immune depressant, had survived. One survives AIDS. But one doesn't survive AZT.

In summary

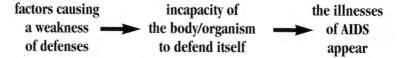

factors causing a weakness of defenses → incapacity of the body/organism to defend itself → the illnesses of AIDS appear

In erasing the factors which cause immuno-deficiency, one prevents and/or cures AIDS. All that seems logical and conforms to common sense. Why then are the authorities upholding, strongly and exclusively, as they have done for the past 10 years, the following formula:

$$HIV + = AIDS = DEATH$$

In making the virus responsible for AIDS, the authorities condemn every person who is seropositive (HIV+), in good health or not, to the diagnosis of AIDS and, next, death. The word seropositive is synonymous with AIDS and it is mixed in with the AIDS statistics. They also have the right to the same murderous and ineffective treatment that is AZT.

While in reality, seropositive means nothing more than having come into contact with the retrovirus HIV. Without immuno-deficiency, no AIDS. One can be seropositive and not lose a wink of sleep!

What is more. This approach, that HIV = AIDS, kills people in good health and prevents those who do have AIDS from recovering. For **AIDS is preventable and can be treated.** But not with AZT. Common sense tells us that it is NOT with immune-depressant medications, which weaken the defense system, that we are going to reinforce the immune system.

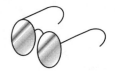

Let us not lose sight of the fact that:

We can choose to live or die. We only have to look at the two approaches of treating AIDS and make a decision. The survivors of AIDS are witnesses to that. Listen to them:

✔ treatment of the illness (war against the virus) with aggressive medications, leads to death.

✔ treatment of the patient (peace of the bodies, soul, spirit) with a reinforcement of his or her immune system, maintains life.

The survivors' recommendation is clear. Take charge of your health and of your life. Consult, become informed, and make your OWN decision.

HIV+ DOES NOT SPELL AIDS

AIDS DOES NOT SPELL DEATH

Why this murderous relentlessness?

Why do the authorities impose by force this idea that:

- AIDS is one, single illness?
- caused by a single virus: the retrovirus HIV?
- is transmitted sexually?
- treated by anti-retroviral medications, powerful immuno-depressants, such as AZT, which precipitate AIDS?
- prevented by practicing safe sex?

Why do the authorities continue to push and recognize only the theory of "HIV alone" as the cause of AIDS? Despite strong opposition to this concept:

- many scientists, led by Peter Duesberg of the University of California, Berkeley. One of the first virologists to study the retrovirus (HIV class). His work resulted in him becoming an elected Member of the National Academy of Sciences. His stance against the medical establishment caused him to be discredited by his profession and lose his research funds.
- Luc Montagnier, of the Pasteur Institute, the official discoverer of the HIV virus in 1983. Since 1990, he states that HIV alone is not sufficient to cause AIDS.
- the evidence of many cases of AIDS without the HIV virus and the many cases of HIV without AIDS.
- the impossibility of one virus being the sole cause, because there are many types of HIV that are secondary to the mutation of the HIV virus.
- the impossibility of proving that the HIV virus causes AIDS. It is however a basic rule of science, that one must establish a relationship of cause and effect between two factors.

- HIV is an inoffensive retrovirus. It can only be activated when the defense system is weakened. In addition, it alone cannot destroy the immune system. Duesberg calls it the pussy-cat. Montagnier says that it needs other factors with it. It seems a far cry from the image of the big bad wolf that it has been given.

- Lauritzen, an analyst in polling research and author of the book, ***Poison By Prescription - The AZT Story*** , which exposed fraud relating to the research, acceptation by the Food and Drug Administration, and the usage of AZT. Which is medically ineffective and dangerous... and, which causes cancer.

- the fierce denunciation of the lying and fraud in the official practice of AIDS treatment. Patients, therapists and journalists angrily blamed the medical establishment at the Convention of Amsterdam. The "survivors" claimed their right to the truth and to life.

The scapegoat virus

As one cannot explain with any certainty the intentions of others, one cannot answer the question: Why do the authorities insist upon killing people? Be that as it may, one can, however, envisage the consequences of the "HIV alone" theory.

1. One has finally found the **perpetrator** of AIDS. The HIV virus. It is much more practical and makes more economic sense to make war against a virus with medications than to tackle and resolve the socio-political problems of drugs, malnutrition, submission, despair. And to stop vaccinations and medications. Moreover, in giving the same name to the virus and the illness, one has created total confusion. Allowing the indiscriminate use of one for the other.

2. One has also found those **responsible** for the epidemic. Homosexuals. Many still refer to it as the "gay epidemic". It is easier to get away with than calling it a "vaccine epidemic". And so, nothing is said about the experimental anti-hepatitis B vaccines received by groups of homosexuals before they had even contracted the illness. Also, the term AIDS has been reduced to the vulgar acronym of STD, Sexually Transmitted Disease, when it is really a question of several illnesses resulting from an immuno- deficiency.

3. One finds the **treatment**. Against a virus, one gives an anti-viral treatment, AZT, which brings in hundreds of millions of dollars for its manufacturers. Close to $700 million in 1991 alone.

4. One finds the means of **prevention**. Safe sex and condoms. One is punished according to our sins. One's morality is saved. And so are vaccines.

5. One finds the **explanation** for the disappearance of the peoples of Africa. Promiscuity causes the sexual transmission of the virus which spreads the illness and brings death to all. It is certainly a much easier answer than saying that the World Bank impoverished them and Saint W.H.O. vaccinated them.

6. One finds an extremely **lucrative** detection and screening **test**. It is so lucrative in fact that protagonists from France and the United States have been battling for some years now to determine which of the two will pick up the royalties.

7. One finds a whole new subject of **research**, which soaks up millions of dollars. But what is one in fact looking for? Imagine the reply. An ANTI-AIDS VACCINE! A vaccine to fight the virus propagated by other vaccines!

8. One finds a new, extremely effective and subtle **tool for population control**, particularly among the poor and non-whites. This policy is not exclusive to the overpopulated countries of the Third World. It also applies to industrialized countries. In its program Agenda for the Eighties. The Trilateral Commission (world government) determined that the ideal, desirable population for the United States would be 100 million people.

9. One finds a means to **limit a person's rights to a private life**. In the name of the rights of the public at large, one divulges the names of people who are seropositive yet in good health. And the names of patients suffering from one or more illnesses of AIDS, patients who are non-contagious. They are pointed out, they are indexed, and what will we do with them? Studies on "seroprevalence", to use a word of epidemiologists, constitute the violation of a person's fundamental rights and open the door wide to another form of genocide. Or the exclusion of "undesirables". Is it by chance that Blacks and the poor are those hardest hit!

The origin of the HIV retrovirus

HIV was officially "discovered" in 1983.

Yet some who have looked at this question, have made astonishing discoveries that have led them to believe that HIV was purely a **laboratory creation** and not the discovery of an already existing virus.

1. In 1982, Robert Harris and Jeremy Paxman published a book entitled ***A Higher Form Of Killing : The Secret Story of Chemical And Biological Warfare*** on the secrets of chemical and biological warfare. They denounced secret experiments carried out on humans by the Army and the CIA during the 1950s. They also reveal the work done by the Army's Department of Biological Warfare at Fort Detrick.

2. In 1985, Robert Strecker, a doctor in gastro-enterology and doctor of pharmacology, concluded that AIDS had been deliberately provoked, be it voluntarily or involuntarily, as a result of testing of the vaccination against hepatitis B on homosexuals. He was also convinced that the African continent had been contaminated in the same way. At the time of the vaccination campaigns against smallpox to study certain effects of bacteria and viruses, at the request of the World Health Organization. He explains that HIV cannot come from nature, as it is so radically different from all other known viruses. It would be the result of a **cloning** of animal viruses, inoculated into humans, which provoked a new illness. Strecker has published a booklet ***Bio-Attack*** and has made a video.

3. In 1987, Alan Cantwell Jr., doctor of dermatology and researcher, reached basically the same conclusions in his book ***AIDS And The Doctors Of Death.***

4. In 1987, Rolande Girard, journalist, wrote of ethnic weapons in her book *Tristes chimères.*

IN 1987, THE WORLD HEALTH ORGANIZATION

OFFICIALLY DECLARED THAT

"HIV IS A NATURAL VIRUS OF UNKNOWN GEOGRAPHICAL ORIGIN".

> **Some Call
> It AIDS:
> I Call It Murder**
> Eva Snead

5. In 1992, Eva Lee Snead, holistic doctor and researcher, wrote two books, ***Some Call it AIDS : I Call It Murder*** and ***the Connection Between Cancer, AIDS, Immunizations, And Genocides***. She stresses the similarity of clinical syndromes between HIV and SV 40, which is present in African green monkeys. The only way that a human can catch SV 40 from a monkey is through physical contact, eating its meat, or by receiving it by inoculation at the same time as a vaccine. It is the same SV 40 that one found in the vaccine Sabin against polio (**"monkey soup" Sabin**) which was used to vaccinate millions of children over the years. Indeed, it has been found that SV 40 causes congenital anomalies, leukemia, cancers, and serious immuno-suppression. **All symptoms similar to those of AIDS**. She establishes the relationships which exist between LEUKEMIA, SV 40, AIDS. For her, AIDS is only another form of leukemia. She demonstrates the responsibility of vaccines in the appearance of AIDS and in the increase of forms of leukemia and cancers.

The saga of AIDS

To put our time-frame in perspective, here is a pot-pourri of dates.

1952: Meeting behind closed doors in Ottawa, Canada, of Canadian, American, and British researchers studying retroviruses.

1959: The World Health Organization warns of the dangers of using vaccines derived from monkeys.

1960: The World Health Organization announces the presence, in vaccines, of unexpected and undesirable viruses.

1960: The presence of virus SV 40 is found in the cell cultures of the African green monkey and one learns that SV 40 WAS PRESENT IN THE MAJORITY OF ANTI-POLIO VACCINES MANUFACTURED FROM LIVING VIRUSES BEFORE THIS DATE.

1961: Vaccination by living viruses begins.

1963: One learns of a tumoregenic virus, which causes tumors, originating from a monkey.

1963: It is reported that the number of cases of leukemia has increased in States where the anti-polio vaccine containing SV 40 was administered.

1963: A biological research program is launched under the auspices of the *Central Intelligence Agency* and the *US Army* at Fort Detrick, in Maryland. It is attached to the National Cancer Institute.

1964: The presence of the virus SV 40 is discovered in children vaccinated against polio with Sabin vaccine.

1964: It is found that viruses of vaccines (living viruses) give malignant illnesses. THE FOLLOWING PROBLEMS OCCUR MORE AND MORE FREQUENTLY AMONG THE GENERAL POPULATION:

   a) deficiencies in the immune system
   b) congenital anomalies
   c) different forms of leukemia
   d) malignant illnesses among young children.

1968: American virologists set up their sophisticated equipment in Zaire.

1969: President Nixon announces his intention to suspend the manufacture of biological weapons and to destroy existing stockpiles.

1969: The beginning of another strong push on cancer research. Retroviruses are in the spotlight because it is known that they cause cancer in animals. Why not also in humans? One quickly succeeds in cultivating these retroviruses on the human cell. One knows how to cancerize human cells. One learns how **to manufacture cancer.**

1970: The World Health Organization and the National Institute of Health decide to inject the virus and the bacteria into children, during vaccination campaigns, so as to conduct a study.

1971: It is proven that SV 40 cancerizes the cells of mice.

1972: The World Health Organization transforms the 1970 study into one focussing on virus which weaken the immune function.

1973: Berg and other leaders in biochemistry reveal the general principles of a new science. **Genetic engineering** is born.

1973: A new retrovirus is isolated: BVV (bovine visna virus).

1974: The hereditary transmission of a foreign gene is a success.

1975: Gallo, an American researcher, announces the discovery of HTLV and states that this virus gives leukemia to certain population groups.

1977: First case of immuno-deficiency. Acquired by a young African woman doctor. Followed by many cases among Blacks, drug users and hemophiliacs.

1978: Vaccination against hepatitis B of homosexuals in New York.

1980: Vaccination against hepatitis B of homosexuals in five American cities.

1980: The appearance of more and more cases of immuno-deficiency which fall into no formerly known categories.

1981: The official debut of the AIDS epidemic.

1983: Official discovery of a retrovirus, which is held responsible for AIDS. It is given the same name as the illness HIV.

1992: "DESPITE 10 YEARS OF THE MOST INTENSIVE AND COSTLY RESEARCH EVER CONDUCTED ON THE SAME ILLNESS, WE ARE ONLY BEGINNING TO REALIZE HOW LITTLE WE KNOW ABOUT AIDS.

THE MOST DISTURBING ASPECT OF THIS OBSERVATION IS THE POSSIBILITY THAT OUR IGNORANCE RESULTS IN LARGE PART FROM THE GREAT FAITH THAT WE PLACED IN THE HIV THEORY.

AS WELL AS THE LITTLE CONFIDENCE SHOWN IN ITS CRITICS.

MOREOVER, EVERY YEAR HAS SERVED TO REINFORCE THE CAUSE OF THOSE WHO PROCLAIM THAT THERE IS MORE TO AIDS THAN HIV.

AND THAT, AS A RESULT, THERE ARE BETTER WAYS OF CONTROLLING AIDS THAN VACCINES, MEDICATIONS, AND PUBLIC POLICIES REGARDING HIV."

Robert Root-Bernstein
Biochemist and immunologist
Professor of physiology
University of Michigan

The trilogy of lies

PART THREE:
Cancer is a mystery

*It is an illness of unknown causes
... or one of the illnesses of AIDS*

A sad statement of account after forty years

After decades of an intensive war against cancer, the situation is the following in industrialized countries:

1. The mortality rate from cancer has increased. More and more people are dying from cancer. Tangible proof that its prevention and treatment are not succeeding.

2. Billions upon billions of dollars have been spent to no avail. "Cancer costs Americans over $100 billion dollars each year... for treatments that are both ineffective and inhumane", reports Frank Wiewel, director of People Against Cancer.

3. The number of deaths continues to grow. Some 500,000 (half a million) Americans die of cancer every year.

4. Millions of people have been tortured. Maiming is commonplace. Nobody escapes it. Patients have to choose between one or more forms of mutilation:

> **"The cancer cure cover-up is America's holocaust."**
>
> Barry Lines

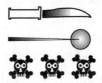

- amputation = surgery
- burning = radiotherapy
- poisoning = chemotherapy.

All these treatments are extremely aggressive. They destabilize the body's organic balance. And seriously damage the immune system.

5. The existence of alternative remedies is either hidden from the public or access to them forbidden. Remedies that are effective, safe and inexpensive. Those who promote them are hunted down. It is like the witch-hunt of the Middle Ages.

6. The rights to **freedom of medical** choice are undermined. Our rights to decide for ourselves, and to determine what we will, or will not do, with our own bodies, have been taken from us.

7. Our immune system has systematically been destroyed by the presence of many carcinogenic products, such as pesticides, vaccines, radiations, medications in the water, air, foodstuffs, and elsewhere in the environment.

Effective treatments since sixty years

On one hand, the authorities continue to have us believe that cancer is an illness that is just as mysterious as it is deadly. And that we must combat it with violence. On the other hand, we know that **effective treatments do exist.** These treatments have existed for sixty years. Could it be that those close to us might still be alive today?

In 1934, in the United States,

Royal Rife and a group of doctors, under the auspices of the University of Southern California, revealed their clinical successes. They had succeeded in destroying the micro-organism responsible for cancer by means of a precise electro-magnetic wavelength. In the years that would follow, the technique of treating cancer using electro-magnetic waves would spread. And many doctors would use it successfully. But not for long.

When Morris Fishbein, director of the *American Medical Association (AMA)*, heard talk of this cancer treatment, he demanded that he be given a part of the action. He was refused. The result of this refusal was not long in coming. Doctors were forced to abandon the new technique. All articles on the treatment in medical journals were forbidden by the *AMA*. Results of this technique obtained by government laboratories were lost. Researchers who supported the treatment, as well as the principles upon which it was based, fell into disgrace and were treated as cheats and liars. The author of the article explaining the technique, published by the Smithsonian Institute, died in a car accident.

Who then was responsible for such a decision? Already, at this time, medicine was for the most part in the hands of financiers. The principal actors defended private interests.

- The all-powerful *American Medical Association*, which issued "seals of approval" on products and medications, in return for remuneration.
- The *Rockefeller Institute for Medical Research*, established in 1902. In 1928, it had already received $65,000,000 in funds from John D. Rockefeller.
- The "king" of microbiology, at this time, was Thomas Rivers, a doctor at the Rockefeller Institute, who in 1926 decreed that viruses and bacteria were two distinct things. He was later director of the Rockefeller Hospital from 1937 to 1955 and vice-president of the Rockefeller Institute from 1953 until his death. His influence on cancer research was significant.
- The *Sloan-Kettering Memorial Cancer Center* in New York, was the first cancer hospital in the United States. It was the medication test centre for large pharmaceutical companies between 1940 and 1955. Interestingly enough, Cornelius Rhoads, after several years at the Rockefeller Institute, was named director of *the Center* in 1939. He remained there up until his death in 1959. He was the biggest defender of chemotherapy in the country.

- *The American Cancer Society*, founded in 1913 by John D. Rockefeller Jr. and his associates, received tons of public money and used it to finance research projects approved by the authorities. Those positions with any decisional powers were held by financial interests.

In the 1950s, in France,

Gaston Naessens, biologist, developed a series of effective anti-cancer products. First GN-24 and then Anablast enjoyed an enormous success, which alerted the authorities. The latter instituted legal procedures. He had to stop treating his patients despite the extraordinary results. In 1964, he emigrated to Canada. There, he developed a new remedy against cancer, 714-X. Again a new success. And a new headline-making trial in 1989. Patients flocked from around the world, all bearing witness to the success of his treatment. The authorities could not condemn him.

> **The Persecution And Trial Of Gaston Naessens**
> Christopher Bird

Whatever the country, the players in the medical system, and their tactics, are the same, to suppress treatments that are effective against cancer. The world financiers and their multinationals are stateless. They have no allegiance. And they exploit all. It is they who control the Medical Mafia in every country. **Donna Governmenta** and her children see to it, on their behalf, that we continue to buy and consume those products which guarantee their profits.

What is cancer?

Cancer is one of the illnesses of AIDS, characterized by disordinate multiplication of cells, which form a tumor. Cancer presents the same symptoms as AIDS: weakness, loss of weight, loss of appetite and fever, caused by a deficiency of the immune system.

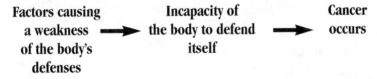

Factors causing a weakness of the body's defenses ➡️ **Incapacity of the body to defend itself** ➡️ **Cancer occurs**

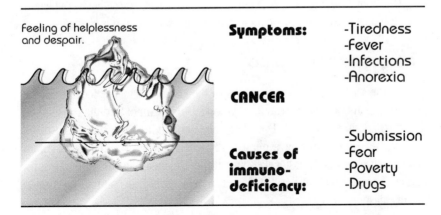

Feeling of helplessness and despair.

Symptoms:
-Tiredness
-Fever
-Infections
-Anorexia

CANCER

Causes of immuno-deficiency:
-Submission
-Fear
-Poverty
-Drugs

Every day, we create a little cancer. Every day, our defense system defeats the tumor. But if our defense system comes to be deficient, it no longer defeats the cancer. It grows and becomes a tumor. This is the **pre-cancerous** phase. The tumor, in turn, secretes a hormone which destroys the immune system.

It wipes it out completely. This is the **cancerous** phase.

What is the cause of the deficiency of the immune system?

The same causes as those for illnesses of AIDS. We saw them in the previous chapter. It is said of cancer that it is sickness of the soul. In fact it is very strongly linked to the emotions. Cancer is often preceded by a depression. The most frequent symptoms are despair and a feeling of helplessness, which reflect the state of our soul. Moreover, patients who come out best, regardless of the treatment, are the fighters, the rebels. Those who refuse to give up.

Bernie Siegel calls them his *"Exceptional Cancer Patients"* in his marvelous book ***Love, Medicine And Miracles*** .

The greatest sickness of the soul continues to be **submission**. To others. To their ideas, their pressures, their fear, their expectations, their laws, their statistics, their treatments.

Let us not lose sight of the fact that:

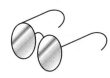

- ✔ cancer is an illness which is treatable and preventable.
- ✔ the principal cause of cancer is to be found in the soul.
- ✔ there is rarely an emergency involved in treating cancer.
  We should take the time to inform ourselves.
- ✔ chemotherapy weakens our immune system.
- ✔ preventing cancer implies reinforcing our immune system.
- ✔ refusing to submit is a plus for a healthy recovery.
- ✔ prognostic are for books, not for human beings.
- ✔ cancer is a wake-up call that we give ourselves.
  Our body is telling us to take the weight off our feet, re-establish contact with ourselves, and re-orient our life. It is a chance that it is giving us.

The scapegoat gene

As for AIDS, the whole question is in the cause of cancer. Because a good diagnosis leads to a good treatment. As long as one cannot find the cause of the illness, one cannot cure it. Even less, prevent it. Since the beginning of the century, the authorities have persistently led us to believe that cancer is an illness that we cannot master. Despite all the evidence, despite all the proof to the contrary, despite all the "spontaneous remissions", despite all the useless deaths, despite...

- In 1974, Norman Zinder, doctor at the *Rockefeller University*, stated: "We do not know how to attack cancer, even less how to conquer it, because we do not know enough about how it works."

- In 1975, the *Sloan-Kettering Memorial Cancer Center* discovered different types of virus-bacteria in the blood of all its patients. But they burned the laboratory results.

Despite everything, the authorities maintain that cancer is due to a **defective chromosome, the cause of which we do not know**. It supports research along this false track. And causes us to hope for the discovery of - what? - a vaccine against cancer!

All this time, people are dying, being assassinated with chemotherapy, radiotherapy, surgery, medications.

And we are being vaccinated in droves.

Better still, we are told of new discoveries about nasty genes and incited to **test our genes** and **submit to early operations to prevent the illness.**

- In April 1994, Time Magazine ran a cover page headline: *HOPE IN THE WAR AGAINST CANCER*. In an in-depth, rather complex and cleverly illustrated article, it praised the virtues of new treatments. For one, a synthetic vaccine. For another, a detection and screening test for inherited genetic defects, which makes us "persons at risk". As such, we have the good fortune of being able to have the operation before the illness appears. **And why don't we have both breasts removed right away?**

That would be real prevention? WHAT MADNESS!

- Lance Liotta, the number one expert in metastase at the *National Cancer Institute*, states: *"After all, we don't cure diseases like diabetes and hypertension. We control them. Why can't we look at cancer that way?"*

- Ann Fagan, 37, having submitted to an ileostomy for a colo-rectal cancer (a bag for cancer of the rectum), and a mother of two girls, is happy for them: "They will have surgical options not available to me. For that reason, I decided they should be tested. I'm a real advocate for early detection."

The reality is that the authorities hid from Ann Fagan the fact that:

- ✔ Her cancer could have been treated differently, without having to resort to a bag. No more than her children will in the future.

- ✔ That there are a lot of other treatments for cancer apart from surgery and chemotherapy. They are much more effective and they have no secondary effects.

- ✔ Cancer is not hereditary. The genetic fault inherited by her daughters probably came from vaccinations.

- ✔ Cancer is an illness which often disappears without surgery, or chemotherapy, or radiotherapy.

> TIME
> **HOPE IN THE WAR AGAINST CANCER**

> **"AIDS is cancer, and cancer is AIDS."**
> Alan Cantwell

✔ Cancer is one of the illnesses of AIDS. That is to say, the **result of an immuno-deficiency**. Those affected with AIDS often die of cancer. Causes of the deficiency of the immune system are known and are treatable, as is cancer.

✔ The only **possible prevention** of cancer, is to maintain the immune system in a healthy state. All aggression, most notably the fear of cancer, is a impediment to that state.

Fatality vs spontaneous remission

The diagnosis of cancer is synonymous with fatality. That is if it is not treated. We are led to believe that it is an EMERGENCY and rush us to have their mutilating treatments. And yet there is no emergency.

Cancer is not an EMERGENCY

Indeed, one should be aware that some patients do not follow the treatments of scientific medicine. And they don't die. More than that, many are cured completely without any chemotherapy, radiotherapy, or surgery whatsoever. The tumor just simply disappears. The experts and specialists are then dumbfounded. For it does not conform to their statistics or knowledge. They therefore conclude that there was a mistake in the diagnosis. "So then why did you propose that I undergo chemotherapy?" asked one patient. No reply.

War on cancer

To confront the plague of cancer, the authorities decided to go all out. In 1971, President Nixon signed the National Cancer Act. It was a declaration of war on cancer.

Waging war is to destroy in the hope that, in the destruction, one also destroys the enemy.

- One thing is certain. One destroys oneself and one's environment.
- One thing is uncertain. The destruction of the enemy.

Who is the enemy?

"Our decades of war against cancer have been a qualified failure."

John Bailar

We are searching for it still! After 40 years of intensive and horribly costly research. Because we have not yet found it. It must surely be well hidden.

Without knowing the enemy, after more than four decades of trying, the authorities continue to **look in the wrong direction**. It is a lot like looking for a rabbit on the same path, day after day, week after week, year after year, decade after decade. Our common sense will tell us that, after a few days, it would be better to look elsewhere if one wants to find rabbits.

But in medicine, science and common sense just somehow do not go together. Nevertheless, certain experts are now beginning to ask questions of themselves.

"We must rethink our basic strategy in the matter of research and ask ourselves whether a new strategy would not be more desirable... if a major re-orientation would not be more advantageous to the public." stated John Bailar lll. A doctor, professor of epidemiology and biostatistics at McGill University, Montreal, Canada, and scientific advisor to the *US Department of Health and Human Resources* in Washington, D.C., he was speaking at the Convention of the FORCTC in 1992 on the epidemiology of cancer.

After 40 years of dismal failures hunting down an unkown enemy, the authorities continue to **strike out in the same manner**. One mercilessly shoots at anything that moves. And with machine guns at that. One amputates, burns, poisons. One destroys everything. Anything goes, in times of war. Fight fire with fire. Anything goes. The enemy must be destroyed. Even if they are still in their cots and have not yet learned to walk. They could grow up to be dangerous. They must be detected early and nipped in the bud. In the name of prevention.

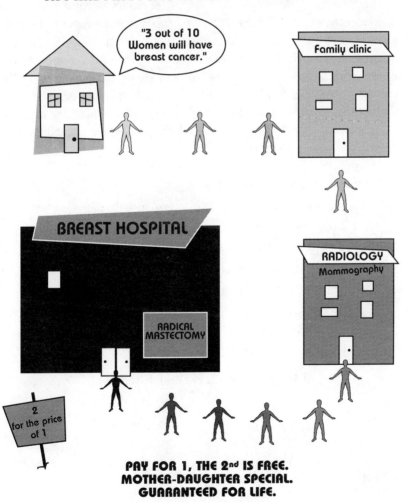

John Bailar went on to add: "I am going to show that this insistence on the progress of treatment represents largely a defeat, and that it is time to seriously consider prevention."

Prevention or early war

Are there two definitions of the word PREVENTION?

To prevent, according to the dictionary, means to make impossible, to keep a thing from happening. In medical parlance, to prevent means to stop the illness from occurring. And to do it in such a way that it never appears.

To prevent is to avoid having to cure.

The authorities, however, use the word prevention in terms of treating the illness as soon as possible. Quite a different usage from the true meaning of the word. When the illness occurs, one treats it. One does not prevent it. As a result, what they call prevention, is nothing more than early detection. The illness is discovered as soon as possible, in order to treat it as soon as possible. This is not to prevent. It is to try to cure it after the fact. As such, it is false representation!

I have a good friend who every year, as a matter of course, goes for a mammogram. Because her doctor recommended that she does so. Two years ago, a suspect test was diagnosed. In addition to having a swollen and very painful breast for the next six months following the examination, she was terribly afraid. Her doctor suggested to her that she participate in a blind test study involving two groups. One that would take a medication. And another that would not. She was so afraid of having cancer, she accepted. She was included in the group which took the medication. You can imagine the rest. She became ill for real!

Let us not lose sight of the fact that:

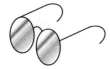

✔ tests called prevention tests are done so as to treat the illness as early as possible.
✔ the equipment is not infallible and often gives false results.
✔ early treatment is to obey the statistics.
✔ passing prevention tests is to bring the sickness upon us.
✔ medicine said to be preventive, more often than not provokes the illness which it tries to avoid.
✔ the only real prevention, is health and peace.

IF YOU WISH PEACE, PREPARE FOR PEACE...
AND NOT WAR.

Cui Bono? The arms merchants

Whenever we do not understand certain policies, which do not seem to make any sense whatsoever, we invariably ask ourselves:*"Cui bono?"* This is the question posed by Ralph Moss in his book, *The Cancer Industry*. This extremely well documented book gives a detailed breakdown of the industry-government liaison, its activities, and what it all means to us.

In English, *Cui bono?* means *who stands to gain?* When we know who profits from a situation, then we known who has created, and who maintains, that situation.

When it comes to war, there is no question that it is the **arms merchants** who gain. It is they who profit. In medicine, these arms merchants, are the manufacturers of weapons used in the war against cancer. Those of chemotherapy, radiotherapy, surgery, and all the hospital industry infrastructure that use and support these weapons. Fraud, lies, conflict of interest, theft, propaganda, control, power play, misinformation. These are but some of the means they use, with no scruples whatsoever, to serve their interests. Even the highly respected cancer societies, such as the *American Cancer Society* in the United States, the *Canadian Cancer Society*, and the *ARC* in France) are part of the plot and continue to get money from us even after we are dead! In making genes the scapegoats for cancer, the establishment of Cancer & Associates:

1. make us believe in the fatality of cancer, in our helplessness in the face of the illness, in our dependence on the authorities and their treatments.

2. distract us from the real causes of the illness. Pollution, poverty, medications, vaccines.

3. deflect all funds for research, treatment, and medications to their own profits.

4. eliminate all competition which could threaten to destroy their financial interests.

And we foot the bill.

But we know that many alternatives do exist to the draconian solutions that are proposed to us by the authorities. Ralph Moss opens our eyes to them in his book, *Cancer Therapy - the independent consumer's guide to non-toxic treatment & prevention.* It makes for fascinating reading.

**The Cancer Industry
- A classic exposé on the cancer establishment.**
Ralph Moss

**Cancer Therapy
- The independent consumer's guide to non
- toxic treatment &
prevention.**
Ralph Moss

...and how about making peace!

Congratulations to all those who have cancer. You are treating yourself to a luxury. You are giving yourself the most beautiful gift possible. For that is the reality. When we say that someone has or is suffering from cancer, we are living an illusion. That illusion is that it implies a sickness, suffering, aging, death. This is not true. In any case, let us take our time. There is no great rush to die as Sandra Ray tells us in her beautiful book *How To Be Chic, Fabulous And Live Forever.*

We have lost FAITH IN OURSELVES. It is to rediscover this faith, that we give ourselves cancer. A marvelous illness, if ever there was one. It causes us to confront death and rediscover our true path in life. At the same time, it affords us the time to make peace with:

💙 ourselves

💙 our family

💙 those around us.

Let us profit from it to rediscover life, health, and peace.

How To be Chic,
Fabulous And
Live Forever.
Sandra Ray

MEDICINE OF WAR	MEDICINE OF PEACE
If you want peace prepare for war.	If you want peace, make peace.
sickness/aging/death	health/youth/life
illusion	reality
nature is fragile	nature is divine
F-P Tandem Fear-Protection	E-E Tandem Education-Empowerment
believing in others	faith in oneself
war on germs, viruses, tumors	peace and ecological harmony
destroys rapidly	reinforces gradually
NONSENSE and (dis) ORDER	COMMON SENSE and ORDER
costly	economical
dangerous	painless
obeying established laws	obeying one's conscience
CONTRARY TO NATURE	**WITH NATURE**

PASTEUR... OR BÉCHAMP?

Two theories

As we can see, there exists two diametrically opposed positions at the core of the medical body. As different as fire and water.

1) Defended by the medicine of sickness, claims that **one unique** agent causes the illness to occur. That agent is an **external enemy** of the body organism. It attacks us and threatens our health.

The germ causes the illness.

It is the **GERM THEORY**. This germ has only one form. And it is always the same. Hence, what is called the **monomorphism** of the germ, **mono** meaning one, and **morphism** meaning form. As a result, the same illness is always caused by the same external agent. And this exterior agent always has the same form. This theory, therefore, in the case of illness, stems from research of the external agent (the enemy) and making **all-out war** on it. It goes even further. It goes to confront the enemy and makes small wars so as to train its troops. Namely, vaccination-prevention. Or to outwit the enemy, surgery-prevention.

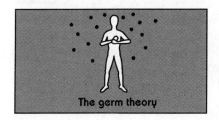

The germ theory

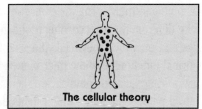

The cellular theory

2) Defended by the medicine of health, claims that it is the body organism itself that manufactures, **inside the cell**, the **different** agents that cause the illness to occur. The agent is an interior friend of the body organism. It tends to re-establish the balance of our ecological system.

The illness causes the germ.

- If its natural environment is disturbed, then it becomes morbid (abnormal, unhealthy) and the illness appears.

- If its natural environment is re-established, it returns to its normal state and the illness automatically disappears.

This is the **CELLULAR THEORY**. A germ may have many forms, depending upon the body organism's state of health. Hence, the **polymorphism** of the germ, **poly** meaning many, and **morphism** meaning forms. As a result, the illness is caused by internal agents of various forms, which become aggressive in certain states of poor health.

Therefore, this theory, in the case of illness, seeks to re-establish good health by all means possible in order to return the germ to its normal state. It re-establishes balance and maintains **peace** between the different elements of the body organism. Health is the prevention of the illness.

Two men

This duality of positions has existed for 150 years. It goes back to the time of Pasteur. And of Béchamp. Both conducted extensive biological research. Only one made the headlines, Pasteur. His name is known worldwide. He symbolizes victory over germs. "Pasteurization" of milk and cheese is an everyday expression. Many hospitals and institutes bear his name. He is famous.

Pasteur is the great defender of monomorphism. **One** germ gives **one** illness. The result of monomorphism is important. It identifies one unique EXTERNAL agent and makes war on it, even if that war depletes the health of the body organism. **The germ is eliminated and the illness disappears.**

As for Béchamp, he worked in obscurity, little concerned about his reputation. He was not known then. And he isn't today. Neither is his name nor his work. No school bears his name. Yet he had an extraordinary microscope which enabled him to identify extremely small corpuscles, even smaller than cells.

These are known as **microzymes** and they are at the very origin of life. They can be found in humans, animals, insects, plants, and micro-organisms. In humans, their form varies according to the person's state of health. They take different forms according to the general condition of the cell in which they live and on which they feed. Illness follows when there is an imbalance in the normal functioning of the microzymes. When the state of health is poor (malnutrition, intoxication, physical or mental stress), the microzyme is transformed into a pathogenic germ which fights the imbalance brought about by the poor state of health.

For Béchamp, the **same** germ may take **many** forms, depending upon the environment in which it lives. But his theory of polymorphism was not endorsed and accepted. The result of polymorphism is important. It is sufficient to reinforce a person's health, for the INTERNAL germs to change back into their microzyme form and reassume their peaceful, protective function. And the illness disappears.

Two systems of values

With Pasteur and Béchamp, it is not only a matter of two different theories. They had two different systems of values. They personify the two fundamental options of our existence on earth:

- external matter or inner spirit
- the enemy germ or microzyme friend
- external power or inner power
- punishment or encouragement
- confrontation or collaboration
- war or peace
- established (dis)order or innate natural order.

Who was right? Ethyl Douglas Hume asked the question and made an in-depth study of the two men. For years, she sifted through the archives and gathered information. Then she published her report in 1947 in a book entitled *Béchamp or Pasteur? - a lost chapter in the history of biology.* In it she takes us back to the time of the two men and goes on...

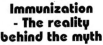

Immunization - The reality behind the myth
Walene James

To about 1850, scientists were speculating about the origin and nature of living matter, and were questioning why milk turned sour, meat rotted, and wine fermented. Where did this phenomenon originate?

The majority of them thought that the "thing" - the living matter - which caused these phenomena came from **nowhere.** It was the theory of "spontaneous generation", very much in fashion at the time. Scientists who adhered to this theory were known as "spontepratists". Pasteur, a chemist, was one of them.

At the same time, another scientist was bent over his microscope studying living blood. He proved that fermentation resulted from **small organisms**, called microzymes, which could be found within the cell as well as outside the body. This man was a chemist, doctor, naturalist, and biologist. It was Béchamp.

Pasteur was ambitious, an opportunist. He was also a genius in the art of promoting himself. And he plagiarized, and then vulgarized, the work of Béchamp. He stole the idea of small organisms being responsible, but he only revealed a small part of Béchamp's discoveries. Pasteur proclaimed that these small organisms only came from the outside. He forgot to mention that, once exposed to air, germs and other morbid (abnormal) microzymes lose their virulence very rapidly. And this deceit has been perpetuated ever since.

Pasteur's fame is particularly linked to his vaccine for rabies. History would have us believe that Pasteur ridded us of this terrible affliction. Yet we know two things.

1. The miracle cure of little Joseph Meister, who was "saved" by Pasteur's vaccine, had nothing to do with being a miracle. It later came out that nobody died, neither the dog who was supposedly infected, nor its bitten master. People who were bitten, and who were not vaccinated, did not die. Those who were not bitten, but who were vaccinated, died from paralysis and not from spasms which are symptomatic of rabies.

2. Rabies, it seems, does not exist. It appears to be an imaginary illness. Dr. Millicent Morden compiled statements by veterinarians and kennel owners in a booklet, *The Fraud of Rabies,* distributed by California Animal Defense and Anti-Vivisection League. According to them, rabies consists of an acute hysterical nervous breakdown. This state is exacerbated by the simple mention of the word rabies, which scares the living daylights out of everyone, specially the one who is sick. Moreover, these "enraged" animals often suffer from hunger and misery. What is certain, however, is that the Pasteur vaccine against rabies produces a state of delirium. What is known as "Korsakoff psychosis," for up to twenty (20) years after the vaccine has been administered.

Pasteur was also famous for the **pasteurization of milk**. This consists of heating it to high temperatures so as to kill the pathogenic bacteria, which cause illnesses, and retard the development of other bacteria. Yet we know that:

1. **The temperature is not high enough**. It requires much higher temperatures to kill the bacteria that give typhoid, coli bacillus and tuberculosis. Some salmonella epidemics have been reported to have come from pasteurized milk. But very high temperatures damage the milk.

2. **The temperature is too high**. It kills the lactic acid which prevents the putrefaction effect of the bacteria. The pasteurization destroys the milk's intrinsic germicidal properties, that is to say its ability to kill germs in the milk. As a result, bacteria multiply much faster in pasteurized milk than they do in non-pasteurized milk. Moreover, pasteurization has a considerable effect on the milk's nutritional value. In this regard, it destroys the enzymes, the principal role of which is to free the nutrients in the food that we eat. For example, almost 50% of calcium contained in milk is not used by our body, if the milk is pasteurized. Despite all this knowledge, however, the authorities continue to pasteurize milk and cheese.

The most recent great assault that the authorities have mounted on our food, and our health, despite widespread public protest, is that of permitting foodstuffs to be irradiated. **An updated version of pasteurization, this time by X-Rays**. It destroys the microzymes themselves, the source of life. Eating irradiated foodstuffs, is eating death!

On his death-bed, Pasteur purportedly stated: "Claude Bernard (biologist) was right. THE GERM IS NOTHING. THE ENVIRONMENT IS EVERYTHING." Unfortunately, there were no journalists there at the time to record his words!

But not two truths

These two theories are diametrically opposed. For Pasteur, it is the germ that gives the illness. For Béchamp, it is the illness which gives the germ. Who is right? Only one. The other is wrong. For there cannot be two truths.

The truth is always in the same place - in common sense. Regardless of the beauty of the theory, it must adapt to reality. And it is that reality that guides us. One only has to see where the theory leads us to determine whether it is true or false. Results do not lie. If they are good, that is good enough for Dr. COMMON SENSE, who we are, to formulate an opinion.

The results of applying PASTEUR'S theory are disastrous. Cancer continues on the rise unabated. It is killing more and more people. AIDS is spreading everywhere. New auto-immune illnesses are constantly appearing. Infectious diseases are coming back with new vehemence. Our health and our money are disappearing before our very eyes. Pasteur's theory leads to war with mutilations of all kinds. Amputations, burning and poisoning associated with vomiting, infections, weakness, hair loss, new illnesses, mutations, and ecological imbalance... DISORDER, SICKNESS, DEATH.

The results of applying BÉCHAMP's theory are marvelous. People re-establish the overall state of their health and reinforce their immune system. Their microzymes return to their natural habitat and resume their normal functions of collaboration. Health returns. Whether it is a question of cancer, AIDS, infectious or auto-immune illnesses, all are curable simply by re-establishing the balance at the very core of the body organism. Béchamp's theory ensures peace, with the re-establishment of inner power and harmony in the organism... ORDER, HEALTH, LIFE.

There is no need of degrees or impressive diplomas and certificates to make a decision. Dr. COMMON SENSE knows that the good theory gives good results. But the GREAT Dr. DOGMA blindly obeys the laws that are taught, despite the evidence. He continues to wage war without respite.

Why this murderous relentlessness?

In order to exploit and dominate.

The decision to continue pasteurizing medicine was taken at a global level, by Saint W.H.O. In order to dominate, submission must be maintained.

Applying the Pasteur theory maintains a practice of medicine of sickness, and generates in us feelings of:

- helplessness vis-à-vis external forces
- dependence vis-à-vis external authorities
- being a victim of other people and events.

There is no domination without submission! Domination allows for exploitation. To the submission, one must also add a little or a lot of fear, according to the degree of hypocrisy, in order to get the victims on the Fear-Protection Tandem. And then lead them as we wish.

ILLNESS PAYS LARGE DIVIDENDS TO THEM

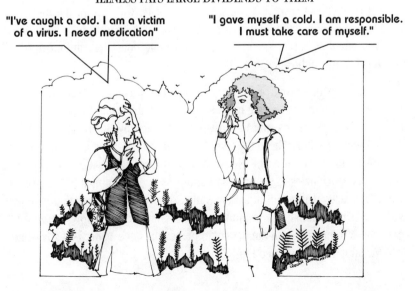

"I've caught a cold. I am a victim of a virus. I need medication"

"I gave myself a cold. I am responsible. I must take care of myself."

Applying the Béchamp theory introduces a medicine of health and generates within us feelings of:

- inner power
- sovereignty. We are the authority capable of healing ourselves
- responsibility (control) for what happens to us.

In addition, treatment of the environment improves not only the health of the individual, but also that of society as a whole. It re-establishes the natural order and with it:

- real equality between individuals.
- equity founded not on laws established by the privileged, but on the legitimacy of the divine right of each and every person
- collaboration
- unconditional love
- prosperity.

HEALTH PAYS DIVIDENDS FOR US ALL

From Béchamp to Naessens

"In a world where everyone cheats, it is the honest man who has the look of a charlatan."

André Gide

The followers of Béchamp have been many. Indeed, history will remember those who have tried to publicly promote his theory. They have all been condemned to silence, either by persuasion, or by force. And since alternative medicines are founded on the cell theory of Béchamp, they too have all but been eliminated and those who practice them ostracized.

For 150 years, the authorities have succeeded, and they are still succeeding, in imposing the **pasteurization of medicine**. Against all common sense and even nature itself. But nature will always have the last word. And woe betide anyone who forgets this!

Throughout my research, a name kept cropping up time and time again. That of GASTON NAESSENS. I soon learned that he was one of the most boycotted scientist of our time. I therefore concluded that he must have been one of the best. For the simple reason that the more one does well, the more one is boycotted by the authorities.

Taking up the work of Béchamp, Naessens pushed it even further. He invented an extremely accurate microscope that enabled him to clearly view not only the small **particles**, the microzymes described by Béchamp, but also all the different forms that they may take. He is able to conclude that illnesses present follow the forms present. He is able to **evaluate** the state of the cell and correct its deficiencies to ensure that the illness does not appear. Real **prevention**. For cases where the illness was already present, he invented a remedy which can re-establish the immune system's good health, allow the germs to come back to normal, and the patient to be healthy once again. Is it any wonder why the authorities boycotted him!

A true answer: the somatidian theory

To the eternal question, "where does matter come from?", the answer is: from the somatid, the microzyme of Béchamp.

The **somatid** is the smallest particle of living matter. It is at the origin of living matter. It is to be found in everything, whether it be animal, vegetable, or human. It can take whatever form, be it spore, bacteria, bacillus. The somatid is the precursor of DNA, therefore of genes. If its capsule is damaged or removed, it is a virus.

The somatid lives unto itself. Placed in a closed jar, without any culture being present, and in total darkness, it grows. **It is life**. The somatid is **immortal**. It is virtually indestructible. As Christopher Bird explains in his book about Naessens: they (somatids) have resisted exposure to carbonization temperatures of 200 degrees Centigrade and more. They have survived exposure to 50,000 rems of nuclear radiation, far more enough to kill any living thing. They have been totally unaffected by any acid.

Upon our death, it becomes bacteria and ensures the decomposition of our organism and its basic components. Namely, oxygen, hydrogen and carbon. Once its job is finished, the bacteria once again becomes a somatid and returns to nature. Naessens told Bird that he would like to examine a sample of moon rock, if only he could, to see if here too somatid forms could be found.

The somatid is an energy condenser. It condenses cosmic energy (Universal, from the Divine Source) and transmits it to matter. It is the link between the spirit (cosmos) and matter. Is that not the definition of SOUL?

A true diagnostic test: the somatoscope

The somatoscope is a microscope which enables ANYONE to see somatids and all their different forms. It is used to look at fresh blood. Blood that is **alive.** It is important to realize that all high magnitude microscopes - electronic microscopes - look at coloured blood. But blood that is **dead**. They are therefore unable to see somatids moving. Thanks to his famous microscope, Naessens was able to describe the complete cycle of a somatid:

- in a healthy environment: somatid spore, double spore, then return
  to somatid. A three - cycle forms.
- in an environment in poor health: the somatid does not change back into
  a somatid after the double spore phase. It enters into a cycle of sixteen
  different forms.

What does that mean in practical terms?

It means that each individual can sit by their practitioner's side and watch their living blood under the somatoscope or on a linked-up television screen. **Each person can see with their very own eyes** the state of their immune system and determine their own state of health. We have this power today. And it is light years away from what is being done today. We are not involved. We do not participate. The state of our health is evaluated by proxy. Figures are provided to us by machines, and transmitted to us by an anonymous voice over the telephone.

With this power, we become our own doctor. We become conscious of, and control, our own state of health. It can be seen. It can be evaluated. We can change it. We can follow its evolution. What's more, every practitioner who knows how to operate a microscope is able to see the somatid in action. All that is required is the addition of a condenser, designed for this purpose, and manufactured so that it can be installed on ordinary microscopes. It is really as simple as that.

A true prevention: improving health

In observing our blood under the somatoscope, we are able to conclude one of three possibilities.

1. our somatid is in a very good state   = good health.
2. our somatid presents some anomalies   = poor health
3. our somatid presents several forms   = illness installed

At stage 2, the illness is not yet installed. If we correct the causes of our poor state of health, we will prevent it and it will not appear. That is true prevention! Let us take the case of cancer, for example. One or two years before the tumor appears, the somatid begins to present anomalies, without always changing form. The tumor has not yet appeared. It is the pre-cancerous stage.

- If we re-establish our health at this moment, the tumor will not appear. If we do not, the tumor will.

It is the cancerous stage. The somatid has entered into its cycle of 16 different forms. The illness is installed. But this is not a sentence of death.

A true treatment: re-establishing health

Once the cancer is established, all is not lost. If one is able to give oneself cancer, one is able to remove it. This is self-healing. One must research and determine the causes of our poor health. With the help of our practitioner, we will analyze different facets of our life on the physical, emotional, mental and spiritual levels. We will correct those that are deficient and lacking. In doing so, we will improve them all. Self-healing is to **correct the cause** of the illness.

This in-depth process may take some time. During this time, we can **rebuild our state of health** and re-establish the good state of our immune system. In order to do this, Naessens perfected a remedy called 714-X. This is injected into the lymph gland and we can learn how to do this ourselves.

There are no side effects. The 714-X does not cure the illness, be it cancer or others. Only we are capable of healing ourselves. But it does rebuild our state of health. Our appetite will improve. And we will regain the strength and energy that we have lost. We are therefore able to correct the very causes of our illness and cure ourselves. If we do not do this, the illness will remain.

The effects of 714-X on one's state of health are easy to see under the somatoscope. Very quickly, after a treatment of three weeks (for cancer), one will already see that the somatid has returned virtually to its normal form. We are therefore able to follow the evolution of our state of health on a regular basis, during and after the treatment.

Choosing between Pasteur and Béchamp

As human beings, we have the **power to choose**. It is that which distinguishes us from animals. The ability to choose is a fundamental right of all. It is also a duty. If we do not exercise our right to choose, we choose not to choose. We choose to let the authorities choose for us.

Let us not lose sight of the fact that the authorities'
choice is motivated by:

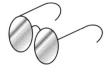

✔ the profits of the multinationals

✔ the performance of the financiers' investment portfolios

✔ reducing the world's population

✔ eliminating those who do not toe the line

✔ eliminating any undesirables (groups or races).

To choose is to take a decision today:

• Continue to leave control of our health to the GREAT Dr. DOGMA

• Or take back control of our health and have confidence in Dr. COMMON SENSE, who we all are.

THE GREAT Dr. DOGMA	Dr. COMMON SENSE
"Every well person is a sick person who doesn't know it." Jules Romains	Every sick person is a God/Goddess who doesn't know it.
medical totalitarianism	individual sovereignty
the germ gives the illness	the illness gives the germ
the powers that be (power OVER)	the power within (power OF)
war on the enemy germ	peace with the microzyme friend
destroy to heal	reinforce to care
NONSENSE and (dis)ORDER	COMMON SENSE and ORDER
sickness/death	health/life
victim/submissive	responsible/all-powerful
react to fear	act with wisdom
established medicine	Mother Nature
PASTEUR	BÉCHAMP

Choosing between Pasteur and Béchamp is much more than a choice of health. It is a choice of life. It is to reply to the fundamental question of our existence:

WHO IS AT THE SERVICE OF WHOM?

To choose Pasteur is to give priority to appearance over essence, to having over being, to matter over spirit. To choose Béchamp is to give priority to essence over appearance, to being over having, to spirit over matter.

Conclusion: do I stop, or go on reading?

THE GOVERNMENT IS OUR ALLY	WE BELIEVED THAT:
We continue to believe that government, its institutions and the entire medical establishment, are concerned for our well-being. A Mafia cannot exist in the health system because we would have known about it long before now and the authorities would have intervened. We cannot doubt or question our leaders. Who would we believe? They may not be perfect, but what would we do without them? Alone, we can do nothing and we would be courting disaster. There is an elite, it is they who have the right to govern and rule. Let us continue to have faith in the authorities. They know better than we do what is good for us. Man is weak and needs to be told what to do. For our own good, let us obey government directives. Because	The system was at the service of the patient.

The system was directed towards health.

The patient was the beneficiary.

The patient was master.

Doctors controlled medicine.

Government served us.

Multinationals were under the control of the government.

Laws protected us.

Insurance companies guaranteed our security.

The authorities saw to our well-being.

We were free. |
| **GOVERNMENT WORKS FOR US** | **ILLUSION** |

CLOSE THE BOOK

(but do not put it away too far,
because we have to get back to it,
sooner or later)

WE REALIZE THAT:

The patient is at the service of
the system.

The system is directed towards illness.

Industry is the beneficiary.

The patient is exploited, dominated.

Doctors have no power of decision
over the practice of medicine.

Government serves the financiers.

Government is under the control of
the multinationals.

Laws control us.

Insurance companies guarantee
nothing but illness and death.

Authorities lie to us and dispossess us.

We are slaves.

REALITY

THE GOVERNMENT IS OUR ENEMY

Just like Colonel "Bo" Gritz of the
American Army, we notice that the
enemy is not outside, but within our
border. A sad observation! We have
been betrayed. We are angry and we
want to cry. But on the other hand, we
are glad to finally see the system for
what it really is, one which is physically and financially ruining us. Let's stop
having confidence in this impostor,
government, which, under the guise of
being a good provider, has betrayed
us in favour of the multinationals and
world financiers. Let's no longer ask
for help, assistance, laws, etc., from
our enemy. Today, we will adopt an
attitude of automatically being
suspicious of all proposals, decisions
or gifts coming from government.
Always look *this* gift horse in the
mouth. If it suggests that we go right,
we will go left. Even if we do not know
why, we will always make the right
decision. Because

GOVERNMENT WORKS AGAINST US

CONTINUE READING

The realization:
self-health

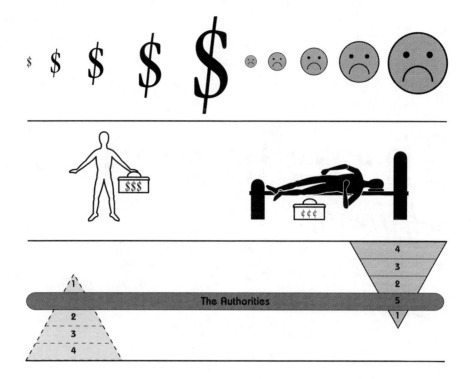

TO LIVE OR DIE?

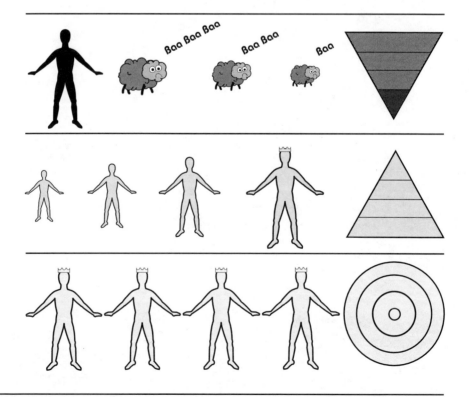

TO RECAPITULATE: before moving on to the realization of our ideal system of health, let us recapitulate what we have seen so far:

1. The **SYMPTOMS**: the medical system:
   - is becoming more and more expensive and is leading to the bankruptcy of countries, regardless of the system and regardless of the country,
   - doesn't suit anyone. Everyone is dissatisfied. Patients and practitioners alike.

2. The **SIGNS**: we note that:
   - all the money goes to sickness, not health,
   - the patient is becoming poorer, while the industry is becoming richer.

3. The **DIAGNOSIS**: the system of health has flipped over:
   - from a system of health, to one of sickness,
   - while conceived for the benefit of the patient, it has become one which benefits industry.

MAKING A CHOICE?

Realizing our ideal system of health involves three stages:

1. The **CAUSE**: finding out why the medical system has overturned
   - the submission to authorities
   - power OVER = external

2. The **TREATMENT**: redressing the medical system
   - individual Sovereignty
   - power OF = inner

3. The **HEALING**: ensuring unlimited, definitive health of the system
   - universal solidarity
   - power WITH = fusion

   In this way, we will re-establish natural order and harmony.

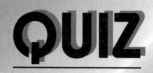

QUIZ

It is often said that "poverty is the mother of all misfortune."
WHO THEN IS THE GRANDMOTHER ?
For the answer, you will have
to turn the book upside down.

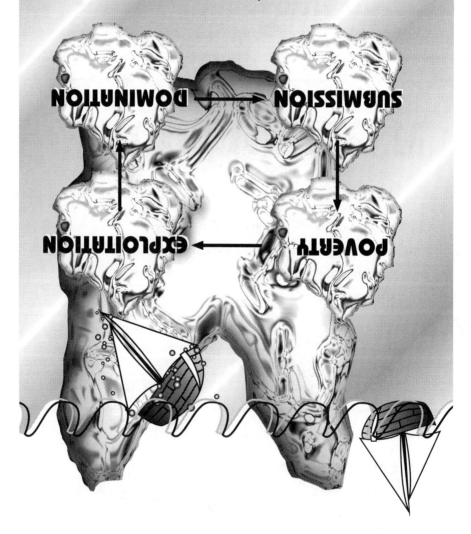

Answer:

Submission

Let us imagine that our boat (the medical system) is sailing between two icebergs in the waters of the far north. One iceberg is named **poverty**. The other, **exploitation**. They appear to us as two distinct icebergs. We are wary of one, poverty, and not the other, exploitation.

Suddenly our boat strikes something and is overturned. Now our head is underwater. And now we can see that the two tips of the icebergs that we saw from above, poverty and exploitation, are twin peaks of the same mountain of ice. **They are the same iceberg!** One could not exist without the other. What affects one, automatically affects the other.

We also notice that the base of the iceberg is huge. That the hidden part (invisible) is much more important than the exposed tips (visible).

We then realize that:

1. **Poverty is the result of exploitation.**
   There is no poverty without exploitation.

2. **Exploitation is the result of domination.**
   There is no exploitation without domination.

3. **Domination is the result of submission.**
   There is no domination without submission.

SUBMISSION IS THE GRANDMOTHER OF ALL MISFORTUNE

Therefore:

1. While **material** poverty is the mother of all misfortune, it is not it that we must attack in order to completely eliminate the cause of capsizing our boat (medical system).

2. It is **inner** submission, the grandmother of all misfortune, that we must remedy in order to be able to navigate in peace.

Knowing this, let us unite all our efforts to **melt the submission.** The melting of domination will automatically follow. Little by little, the tip of exploitation will disappear, as will that of poverty. We can then right our boat and from then on sail safely and peacefully on the seas without striking any obstacles.

For the rest, you will have to turn the book, again.

SELF-HEALTH

Self-health is personal management of health. In order to do this, we must take back complete control of the financing of our health. We must also recognize our total responsibility in the face of whatever happens to us. **Self-health is not possible without self-sickness**. We alone are responsible for the present state of the system. We alone can put it right.

The taking back of control over our health will automatically also free practitioners from the shackles of the present system. This will allow them to practice the medicine of health that they judge to be the best and, in doing so, better serve their patients.

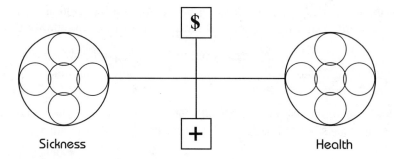

Sickness   Health

THE CAUSE OF THE CAPSIZING: SUBMISSION

In order to realize what we have to do, we must first know the root of the problem. The cause of the overturning of our system of health is our SUBMISSION. Whether patients or practitioners, we have all abandoned our sovereignty. We have given it to the authorities and are submissive to them. We must now be obedient and loyal to them. We have traded our inner power for illusions. Namely, security and protection.

As we have seen at the beginning of this book, submission is the primary cause of all sickness. It is the sickness of the soul. It affects all the bodies. It is at the origin and root of the vicious circle of sickness. It engenders fear, obliterates the conscience, and creates poverty.

To accept submission is to	*To exercise one's sovereignty is to*
• accept slavery	• choose freedom and life
• accept sickness and death	• rediscover health
• accept the priority of the body over the soul	• re-establish the priority of the soul over the body
• accept that the spirit is at the service of matter	• choose that matter is at the service of the spirit
• accept an overturned system	• right the system

Scientific medicine, the tool of submission

As we have noted, illnesses are first and foremost social in nature. But scientific medicine has made us believe otherwise. But how?

Medicine said to be "scientific" has its origins in **SCIENTISM**. This doctrine consists of only recognizing that which can be measured and evaluated in numerical terms. It denies anything that is invisible, including thoughts, emotions, intentions. It limits the Universe to the visible world. And its functioning to that of physico-chemical reactions. That which it cannot see and measure simply does not exist. Figures are everything.

- The human body becomes equated with a machine, different parts of which may be treated independently without affecting the body as a whole.

- Human beings become entities with no relation to their physical, psychological and social environment.

- Practitioners become technocrats who use statistics learned by rote, and apply them to the letter.

In this way, the social context of problems becomes irrelevant. Once the social context is set aside, then everything may be quantified in terms of figures, norms and statistics. One can treat the figures. Common sense and initiative are no longer prerequisites for technocrats. They are replaced by bureaucrats and computers. The machines decide.

The advantage of this scientific doctrine, as Berliner so aptly explained in 1975, is that it transforms problems of a social origin, for which the solution is political, into "scientific" problems, for which the solution is technological. For example, violence which stems directly from social injustice. "Violence begets violence". The problem is social. Yet to master it, scientific justice increases its electronic controls and the efficiency of its police. And everyone is reassured, while the violence continues and our dollars disappear. This is how scientism has avoided the embarrassing social problem created by exploitation and has substituted a technological solution.

SCIENTIFIC MEDICINE was inspired by this doctrine to apply the same criteria to medicine. In this way, it can reject the social causes of illness. And avoid treating poverty, the mother of all misfortune.

Every social problem has been replaced by a scientific illness with a techno-logical solution. For example, poverty causes underweight babies to be born. Scientific medicine provides these babies with a scientific solution, involving incubators, medications, etc. It has even created a special discipline in this regard called neonatality. It can therefore avoid the real problem, which is poverty. Why is there still poverty in our country of such abundance?

Even hygiene, and we know how important that is to health, has quietly taken a back-seat to the profitability of vaccines. Every illness has its own vaccine! Even research neglects the importance of social factors which contribute to sickness. For years they have been searching, and we are still all impatiently waiting, for a vaccine against cancer and another against AIDS. When we know that it is vaccines themselves that cause these illnesses!

Scientific medicine is not scientific

In order to impose scientific medicine, one has established a doctrinal system. And everyone is forced to adhere to its tenets:

- Medical students are selected based on their scientific performance, as well as their loyalty and blind submission to the goals and ideals of scientific medicine.

- University education, the stage prior to medical school, teaches that science is limited to the concrete (that which can be seen and touched) and denies the abstract (that which cannot be seen or touched).

- Authorities impose by force, that is to say by obligatory scientific proof, the scientific practice of medicine. And they forbid all other practices, particularly that of alternative medicines.

Yet scientific medicine **has not been proven scientifically!**

- In 1978, the *Office of Technology Assessment* conducted a major study on scientific medicine and presented its results to the Congress. It concluded that 80% to 90% of treatments used in scientific medicine have not been proven by clinically-controlled studies. In other words, they were being used and taught extensively despite the fact that they were not scientifically proven.

- In 1985, the *National Academy of Science* repeated the same study. With the same results.

It is a simple matter of arithmetic to determine that no more than 10% to 20% of all treatments used in scientific medicine - make that said to be scientific - have been proven by clinically-controlled tests. This means that **the vast majority of medical treatments have no scientific basis whatsoever!**

Scientific medicine is a system of belief

- Either one believes in it and is on the right path,
- or one doesn't believe in it and is a heretic.

Like a religion, it establishes its arbitrary doctrine and demands blind obedience. As in all systems of belief, those who contest it are declared to be heretics. The "non believer" doctor is accused of practicing a medicine that has not been proven scientifically. Therapists are accused of illegally practicing medicine. In one case or the other, the result is the same. **Beat the insubordinates into submission or suppress them** so that the privileged may maintain their privileges.

Scientific medicine makes one ill

It causes iatrogenic illnesses. These are illnesses created by medical intervention. For anyone who would like to read a well-documented study of the present system of health, I highly recommend **Medical Nemesis** by Ivan Illich. It is a small, inexpensive book that is easy to read. In it, he describes, among others, three types of iatrogenic illnesses:

- **clinical:** illnesses caused by the doctor
- **social:** illnesses created deliberately by the machinations of the medical-industrial complex
- **cultural:** illnesses of stress which sap the will of patients to survive.

Scientific medicine alienates patients.

Scientific medicine is in the pay of the financiers

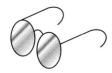

Let us not lose sight of the fact that:

1. Scientific medicine was established by financiers. The Flexner Report was financed by the Carnegie and Rockefeller Foundations.

2. It was spread by them. Abraham Flexner was hired as Secretary of the Board of Directors on Education of the Rockefeller Foundation to implement the recommendations of his report everywhere.

3. The Declaration of Alma Ata, which consecrated the "world ministry of health" of Saint W.H.O., was co-sponsored by the World Bank and the Rockefeller Foundation.

> Tell me who pays you and I will tell you who you serve...

4. Foundations of all kinds continue to support medicine. Financing from foundations consists of combining their money (that of our exploitation, as well as their tax evasion) with public funds (our taxes) for projects of a humanitarian nature. Projects determined by the foundations themselves to serve their own goals. The bottom line is that we finance projects serving the interests of financiers. While they reap the benefits and all the prestige.

5. The financiers are owners of pharmaceutical and technological industries which supply scientific medicine. All have a vested interest in us being sick and that we take drugs.

> **"Profit**
> **x**
> **philanthropy**
> **=**
> **control."**
>
> Gary Allen

6. The financiers control the governments of countries and, by the same token, the laws and the finances of their health systems. With no obstacles at all in those countries where health systems are socialized.

7. The financiers are responsible for social injustice, poverty, violence and the illnesses that result. It is in their interest to see that social sicknesses are replaced by scientific sicknesses with technological solutions.

This is why the medicine of sickness continues to ravage populations of the world. This despite its exorbitant cost and widespread discontentment.

The punishment for insubordination

It has been true throughout the ages. Refusing to submit to the authorities, insubordination, has been severely punished. Most of us only have to go back to our school days to know that it was always the rebellious ones who were on the receiving end of the stick.

> **"If the world can be saved, it will only be by the rebellious."**
>
> André Gide

Just try to go against the flow, the established order, in any profession. There is a high price to pay by those who disobey the authorities and their laws. The same is true in medicine. Doctors and therapists who propose or recommend to their patients different approaches, therapies or solutions, other than those imposed by the authorities are punished. It's totally immaterial if these:

- have helped us: they are punished
- comply with our request: they are punished
- avoid us complications: they are punished
- have improved our health: they are punished.

Who punishes?

The authorities. The Medical Mafia. Either directly, or through the intermediary of family members. They work very closely together. This is why one often finds them working as a team on the same "case", comprising medical, fiscal, judicial, law enforcement members. It is difficult to escape their inquest. Once they cast their net, the catch is guaranteed.

Why do they punish?

To defend the interests of the multinationals. That is to say to ensure the sale of the greatest possible number of vaccines, drugs and technological equipment. In order to do so, they must encourage and create illness everywhere and for everyone. Faithful to this directive, our medical and political authorities make sure that it is applied on a national scale. The W.H.O. and the multinationals do this on a global scale. **Beware all those who oppose them!** The entire Medical Mafia will combine forces to make sure that they understand and "come to their senses".

How do they punish?

The same as they did during the Inquisition in the Middle Ages. With a good old-fashioned **witch-hunt.**

- they hunt down the quarry
- they dispossess it of its belongings and rights
- they torture it and, finally
- they sacrifice it.

Just like during the Inquisition, the sooner the victims give up, the sooner the torture ends.

Hunting down the quarry

1. **Fear**, the silent threat.

   It is the weapon "of choice" to prevent insubordination. We only have to know what awaits us, and what has happened to others, for the authorities to keep us obedient and docile. Fear ensures 'omerta', the code of silence. You think that your doctors are strong and brave? They are human beings just like you. They are just as much afraid of the authorities as you are, if not more so. I have seen doctors working in the top ranks of the medical hierarchy kowtow to their superiors. A title or diploma does not necessarily instill valor.

2. **Intimidation**, the threat of a threat.

   The authorities operate in a decorum of power and secrecy. They write letters menacing their very bosses, the "guilty" doctors and admonish them from their lofty perch. Everything they do is designed to make the quarry feel small and guilty, without them ever knowing what ultimate fate awaits them.

3. **Harassment**, the ongoing threat.

If the quarry hasn't yet given up, harassment is used to make it understand the error of its ways. From simple reprimands to formal warnings. They are dragged from one committee to another. From one court to another. They had better wise up and act accordingly. Or else! The objective of this technique is to wear them down, both physically, morally and financially.

4. **Shame**, the open threat.

The shame felt by a practitioner being pursued by the authorities is similar to that felt by a victim of aggression. It is the victim who feels ashamed, while it should be the aggressor. To increase the pressure, the authorities point the finger of shame through the media.

5. **Ridicule** which, as one proverb says, kills.

The authorities know this full well and do not hesitate to use it to their own ends. One only has to ridicule a treatment technique, a simple phrase or act, or even a physical characteristic of a person, to rob it of all value.

Such was the case, for example, with Jacques Benveniste, a doctor researcher recognized at VINSERM in France. He was visited by a team of observers when he was conducting a scientific study of his famous discovery of the memory of water. This study shows beyond all doubt the effectiveness of homeopathy. So that no one would miss the point of the visiting team's bias, they brought along a magician!

6. **Doubt**, which saps credibility.

It is a very subtle art which causes us to abandon our powers of reasoning and common sense when confronted by someone or something. One only has to sow the seed of any kind of lie, without exactly spelling it out in words, for some people to lose faith in their own opinion. And, in doing so, come to accept that of the authorities.

7. **Diversion**, sowing confusion.

This too is a subtle weapon often used to confuse the quarry. It distracts its attention from the authorities' main objective. For example, how doctors fill out their medical files has become an often-used ploy when the authorities cannot find anything more serious to go after. As if the way a file is filled out influences the practice of medicine or the well-being of the patient!

8. **Labeling**, closing the mind.

The label that is most often used to punish medical insubordinates is that of **charlatan**. As soon as we hear the word charlatan, we freeze. Our mind snaps shut like a giant clam. And we just don't want to hear anything more about it. This is the very purpose of labeling. To shut down the conscience and prevent valuable information from reaching it. The word **placebo** has exactly the same effect. It too saps the marvelous effects of homeopathic remedies.

9. **Defamation and slander**, the shotgun approach.

This is the big gun in the punishment arsenal. The entire Mafia is on the alert and lashes out in all directions. It is used in cases of extreme defiance where it is necessary to completely destroy the quarry, quickly and by any means possible. The threat is too great to allow for the sport of a good hunt. Few can stand up to this sort of punishment. Those who do resist pay dearly.

The quarry is dispossessed of its rights and belongings

10. **Dispossession of its rights.**

The most frequent example is that of the right to practice. It is either withdrawn or suspended. Sometimes, this is even followed up by the dispossession of another basic right. That of freedom. The quarry is carted off to prison. All this is done according to the rules of the art. Arrest by the police, search and seizure, a trial, defamation in the newspapers, prison. The route is all mapped out.

The most commonly used accusation varies according to who is being hunted down.

- If it is a doctor, he or she is accused of practicing a medicine, which is **"not based on scientific proof"**. Bear in mind the reports which found that only 10% to 20% of all scientific medicine treatments were proven to be scientifically effective.

- If it is a therapist, he or she is accused of **"illegally practicing medicine"**. Yet these are not strictly medical treatments, because one also condemns doctors for practicing these same so called NON-medical treatments. Go figure...

The authorities will not let anything deter them from their goal. No **absurdity**, lie, or any other craziness.

In losing their right to practice, practitioners also lose their clientele, their livelihood, and their reputation. Their careers are ruined.

11. **Dispossession of its belongings.**

In general, a fine is imposed. But the financial penalty can also take quite another form. And here again, the Mafia connivance between the medical establishments and its associates is very evident. The weapon is fiscal control.

The tax "man" suddenly shows up. Can you imagine a more effective means than that of an audit? Resulting, as always, in a loss of time, energy and money for the unfortunate victim.

It is such an effective weapon that the medical authorities have adopted it with another slant. The health insurance companies "check" doctors' past billings. The fate of the victims is then placed in the hands of a committee which arbitrarily sanctions the terms of the reprimand and the amount to be repaid. It is often too expensive to appeal the decision before the courts as the victims have to pay their lawyers from their own pockets, unlike the authorities who use our tax money to do so.

One tortures the quarry

12. **Violence**.

For those who have not yet "cried uncle", there are other more drastic means in store. Their laboratories, or their research funds, are taken away.

 Such was the case of Duesberg, an American doctor and eminent researcher in immunology, for having stated, and for continuing to do so to this day, that the HIV virus is not responsible for AIDS.

And as if that wasn't enough, their laboratories and products are destroyed. The sale of their remedies or equipment is forbidden, by having them declared as illegal.

 This was the case with Rife, a biologist who invented a piece of equipment to treat cancer, and who refused to hand over a financial share in the discovery to the then president of the American Medical Association. In response to that refusal, the latter forbade all doctors from using this marvelous invention. If they did so, they would lose their right to practice.

The quarry is sacrificed

13. **Putting it to death.**

Alive or dead, the quarry has been bagged. It can no longer be a nuisance to the interests of the multinationals. In general, by this time, it is totally exhausted. If not, it will be given the *coup de grâce*. The authorities will stop at nothing to hammer the insubordinate into submission. Remember, these are the same authorities that killed thousands during the Opium Wars, in order to ensure the sale of their drug. Today, it is still a question of drug sales. Even if they are legalized, they are no less deadly. And they are still very profitable.

In conclusion, let us not lose sight of the fact that:

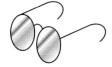

✔ those who only wish us well are condemned as charlatans.

✔ the real charlatans, the mafiosi of health, enjoy their freedom and privileges.

✔ the lack of concern on the part of patients, doctors, journalists, jurists kills us and impoverishes us all.

LET US APPLAUD ALL THOSE WHO THE AUTHORITIES CONDEMN

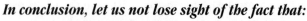

> **Racketeering in Medicine
> - The suppression
> of alternatives**
> James Carter

The story of the cat and the mouse

Recently, I was reading about James Carter, M.D., Dr. P.H., who had exposed details of this situation in his book entitled ***Racketeering in Medicine - The suppression of alternatives*** . Despite the horror stories that he described in his book, I couldn't help but smile. It reminded me of my childhood when the family cat would stalk and catch a mouse and then eat it in front of my grandmother. My poor grandmother just couldn't stand it. She found the scene simply horrific and would always shudder. Much to the amusement of we children.

The cat chases the mice, catches them, plays with them for as long as it amuses it, and then **invariably** ends up **eating** it. It is exactly the same scenario in medicine. The cat always wins. The mouse always loses. It is **medical terrorism** on the part of the cat. Perhaps it is time that we changed the story.

Shortly after reading Carter's book, a group of practitioners invited me to speak to them about fear. Notably the fear of harassment and of reprisals by the medical authorities against practitioners of holistic medicine. My story of the cat and the mouse came back to me. I related it to them and, together, we set out in search of creative solutions to put an end to the despotic rule of the cat.

The cat's offensive

Q. Who are the mice?

A. Every doctor, therapist, healer, or healthcare worker who practices a medicine other than the scientific medicine, sanctioned by the authorities.

Q. Who is the cat?

A. Scientific medicine. Carter calls it "**organized** medicine". Would this be that organized by the Medical Mafia? He calls it the medico-pharmaceutico-industrial complex, which he defines as a "vast mosaic of special interest groups which exercise a disproportionate influence to maximize profit and perpetuate the status quo in the fields of medicine." It is precisely the **Medical Mafia.**

Q. Why does the cat eat the mice?

Because it is hungry? Because of voracity?. Because they taste good? Because that is all they know?

If it is because of hunger, let's simply feed it.

If it is because of the taste, let's simply manufacture synthetic mice that smell and taste just like the real thing.

If it is because it doesn't know any better, let's educate it.

A. It is voracity. The cat's insatiable need for power, money and prestige, constantly commands it to eat mice. It is power crazy!

Q. How many mice can a cat eat at once?

One at a time? Several? All at once?

If it is one at a time, let's choose the toughest.

If it is several at a time, let's give it indigestion.

A. One at a time. Two at the most. It derives just as much pleasure from torturing the mouse as it does from eating it. It is in no hurry to end the torture. That is part of the fun of it. It also instills fear in the other mice to keep the others in line. Each mouse tries to be as discreet and invisible as possible so as not to draw the attention to itself and end up as the next snack.

Q. How can the cat succeed in eating all the mice?

A. The cat is intelligent and lazy. It is therefore cunning. It knows how to **divide and conquer**. It has learned that if it is going to dispose of all the mice, then it must do so progressively, let them fight among each other, and then simply finish off those who are left over. The really big ones.

- It gets all the **big** mice (medical experts, specialists, professors) on its side and gives them privileges, power and prestige, to dispose of the smaller mice. The poor things don't realize that one day they too will just be another snack.

- It manages and controls the **medium-sized** ones (doctors) by giving them advantages that other mice do not have. Better hours, better meals, better living conditions, better terms, better insurance. They are very afraid of the **big** mice and so they obey. The poor things do not realize that they too are on the menu!

- It leaves the **little** mice (therapists) to their fate and the greed of the other mice. It encourages the **medium-sized** mice to invade their territory, pick from their dish, and take the food from their mouths.

Whatever their size, the mice don't realize that **all will be eaten, sooner or later**. They do not see the cat's strategy and they fall into its trap.

The defense of the mice

Faced with the threat of imminent extinction, the mice band together and draw up a strategy of survival.

1. Stop being **afraid**. Fear paralyses the conscience and prevents the mice from seeing what is actually happening, thinking and acting. It is the worst adviser of all. The mice must always remember that cats which use fear are the very ones that are most vulnerable to fear.

2. Rid the cat of its **appetite** for mice. Steps that make eating mice a most unpleasant experience include:

- Attack the cat with an **army** of mice ready to bite on all sides whenever it begins to threaten any mouse. In order to achieve this, the mice must stop waging war between themselves, become organized, draw up their plans in advance, and stick together no matter what happens. They must be ready to intervene in strength at the very first sign of aggression.

- Give the cat **indigestion.** Put pressure upon it from all sides. From citizen's committees for freedom of choice in terms of therapies, newspapers, other doctors, politicians, lawyers. Everyone should be made to understand why the mice are savagely attacked. And why the cat must be stopped.
- Make sure that eating mice **leaves a very bad taste** in the cat's mouth. The cat always uses intimidation and makes the mice feel ashamed so as to weaken them before it strikes. If that is to stop, the mice must turn the tables. They must denounce in a loud and clear voice the abusive power of the cat.

To better understand shame, put yourself in the position of a woman who has been battered by her husband. She feels shame and suffers in silence. But the day she speaks out and denounces what is happening, she gives this shame back to her husband. It is now he who becomes ashamed, as it should be.

- The mice must make it known publicly that only they serve the truth and freedom of choice while the cat serves a system that is entirely based on secrecy. That 80% to 90% of the so-called "scientific" medicine imposed by the cat is not scientific at all. The mice must also show that what the cat is doing goes against all scientific principles and is harming patients.
3. Hold the cat at bay. Team up and **make an alliance** with a large watch-dog (the media). Work closely together. By informing it of the cat's antics, it can alert the public of the danger. The cat will never dare indiscriminately attack a mouse again in the presence of a dog with teeth.

General peace - the end of the story

The mice put up such a co-ordinated and effective defense that they beat the cat. The cat leaves home. The mice throw a great party and celebrate. They have won the battle. But, unfortunately, not the war.

The very next day, however, another cat shows up. Even more fierce than the one that has just left. Only then do the mice realize that cats are in the pay of an **invisible master**. They also realize that fighting is not the solution.

For several days, the mice scamper about the house searching in vain. They do not find whoever is responsible for giving the cats their orders. He remains hidden away in his headquarters somewhere else in the world. He is unreachable. He is a member of a worldwide organization dedicated to the extermination of mice.

Suddenly, a mouse cries out. It has just found a bound and gagged lady in a closet. The mice all rush and free her. They ask her: "Who are you?" **"The mistress of the house"**, she replies.

The mice tell her of their misfortune. She listens to them attentively and comes to understand that they, and she herself, have been victimized by the same invisible impostor. He had imprisoned her, passing himself off as the master of the house. And in this way, he was able to establish his rule. And create war and disorder in the very heart of the home.

She explained to the mice that her name was **"Patient"**. And that she was the sovereign of the house. Now that she was free, she would reassume the control that she once had and re-establish order. And so she did.

The mice came to understand that only the **"Patient"** had the power to re-establish order. And from now on, they would work together to protect forever "her" sovereignty. And order and peace returned to the household. From that day on, all lived in peace and harmony under the very same roof.

The moral of this story

The first lesson to be learned is that patients are the true sovereigns of the health system. **Only they have the power to remedy it**. Not doctors and certainly not government.

The second lesson is that the false and bogus masters of the medical system are hidden far away from us. These are the inaccessible world bankers who control through their go-betweens, **the authorities do their beckoning.**

The third lesson is that the authorities are afraid of journalists and that journalists are looking for true and valid information and news. Let us give it to them. The authorities get away with any lies they wish to plant with the media. Journalists will not know the truth if we do not give it to them. Let us establish **close and permanent ties with journalists** in all facets of the media, both print and electronic.

The fourth lesson is that practitioners should stick together. There should be no **hierarchal** distinction between surgeons, specialists and general practitioners. Also between doctors and non-doctors, either working in hospitals or anywhere else. Let us replace competition by collaboration. And let us stop stealing from one another's plate. Particularly when one already has more than one's fair share.

The fifth lesson is that **only love** can lead to peace and life. Any kind of battle, whether offensive or counter-offensive, automatically leads to war and inevitable death. Let us end our submission to fear and exercise our individual, all-powerful sovereignty of Love and prosperity.

Power OVER, power OF

Power is the fact of being able to. That is to say of HAVING the ability, the right, the strength to act. TO BE in a state of, TO BE capable of, to have the faculty, the possibility of doing.

Power may be exercised over **others:**

- It is the power OVER their destiny
- It is HAVING power over others
- It is dominating and exploiting
- It is a win-lose game.

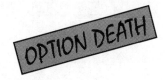

The power OVER is based on illusion. Those who play it are like those who play "Monopoly". But around a board that is on a world scale. And like those who **forget** that it is more than just a game. That the pieces, houses, hotels, dice and money are nothing more than an illusion. They fight all out, to the death as it were, just to win. Just for the sake of winning, for the money is not real. Their power OVER others is dependent upon others whom they must control in order for they themselves to be powerful. They know only victory and defeat. Sooner or later, they will succumb to the game.

Power may be exercised over **oneself**:

- It is the power OF one's destiny.
- It is the power of BEING oneself.
- It is creating equality and equity.
- It is a win-win game in which everyone comes out a winner.

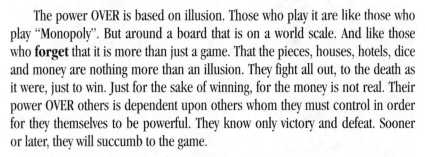

The power OF is based on reality. It is innate. Everyone has it. Everyone is a winner. It does not depend upon others. It is sovereign. All-powerful. Eternal. It is of divine nature.

POWER OVER	POWER OF
Power established by the privileged to maintain their privileges	Power that is inherent to each individual to realize their destiny
patriachal	Mother-Nature
established	innate
outside oneself	inside oneself
relative	absolute
limited	unlimited
human	universal-cosmic-divine
rights established by man	divine Universal Right
acquired by legality	based on legitimacy
the laws of man	Universal laws
imposed by fear	realized voluntarily
taught by obedience	promoted by dignity
leads to dependence	leads to autonomy
encourages irresponsibility	favors responsibility
domination and possession	helps others and shares
SUBMISSION to authorities	SOVEREIGNTY of the individual
it is slavery	it is freedom
ESTABLISHED (dis)order	**NATURAL order**
SUBMISSION	**SOVEREIGNTY**

Being power crazy: the control syndrome

Once again, I am going to make an abstraction from our normal way of thinking and walk in the shoes of those in power. For **us**, power means the ability to do something. To accomplish a task. To overcome a challenge. That is the **POWER OF**.

For the **Godfather**, power consists of controlling others, imposing his law, and dominating them. That is the **POWER OVER**. In order to achieve this, he must have more money than the others. He must always have the advantage. The edge. He will never have enough because someone may always have more than him. In order to keep potential rivals in line, and under his control, he will give them control over others. And they, in turn, will do the same to others. This is the pyramid of power. Everyone strives to reach the next rung of the ladder and, in doing so, have the greatest possible power over others. Those who are still climbing. It is an insatiable game. It is crazy. As is being power crazy.

People who are afflicted with this sickness are insecure. They hide their insecurity by exercising control over others. The more they are insecure, the more despotic, the more tyrannical, they become. The higher they climb on the ladder of power, the more dissatisfied they become. They spend half of their life accumulating money and power. And the rest hanging on to it. Protecting it, so as not to lose it. What a miserable way to live!

Control or
be controlled

- Such people know only war. Control or be controlled. Win or lose. Of the two options, their choice is understandable. They always want to win. And to win more and more. If they are to achieve this, they must always control. More and more people. It is a vicious circle. Whenever one plays the role of torturer one day, one cannot forget that one will be a victim the next. The two roles alternate.

- Such people do not know peace. Paradise on earth for all. They don't even know that it exists. They are prisoners of their thoughts and of their fears. They cannot even peek through the gate of their prison to see the shining light behind. They have submitted to fear and are prisoners of it.

Anyone who lives in submission of fear and of preconceived ideas is like them. Like them, believes in elitism. In maintaining the social hierarchy. And in preserving the concept of domination and exploitation.

We are all sometimes, in our own way, controllers or someone who is controlled. We are all torturers or victims. The only thing that differentiates us from them is our degree of craziness. They believe that they have power over us. We believe that they have power over us. We are both crazy. They because they are prepared to sell their family, their children, their loved ones, their soul, to win the game. And we because we dedicate all our energy to defending ourselves against them. Whether attacking, or defending, it is game of war. And a deadly one at that!

Are we all crazy without knowing it? And could those who are said to be crazy because they refuse to join our craziness really be sane?

Medical control

The same hierarchy of craziness rules the medical field. Government has usurped the power of patients in promising them security. The patients believed it and entrusted their money to government not knowing that it would be given to industry. This is a very poor beginning. How do we get out of the trap?

... BY BECOMING AWARE:

- of the patriarchal, social hierarchy in which we live. It is a system that is supported and maintained by a minority in order to control the majority. By making us argue and fight between ourselves. "Divide and conquer!" Stop being used like this. **Let us replace competition with collaboration.**

- that by giving up our financial power (for our security) and our medical power (for our protection), we lose our rights. Our supreme power. Nobody has the right to decide for us. **Let us replace submission to the "authorities" with our sovereignty as clients and employers.**

- of our non-caring attitude and of our inertia (transfer of responsibilities) when confronting everyday problems that have allowed the authorities to wedge themselves between doctors and their clients. We are all responsible for ensuring that the system works well and that it is accessible to all. **Let us replace irresponsibility with responsibility.**

- that uncertainty drives us even further apart and gives rise to poverty and violence. **Let us replace possession with sharing.**

- that elitism is an exploitation tool of the privileged that serves to let them control the majority. **Let us replace our so-called leaders with our own inner power, our sovereignty.**

- that any law, whatever it may be, is an infringement on our freedom. Everyone is born sovereign with all inherent rights. It is the unlimited legitimacy of Universal Rights. The privileged have created legality, their own law, which they impose upon us to eliminate our legitimacy. **Let us replace legality with legitimacy.**

- that silence is golden only for the authorities who exploit it, and us, with our tacit consent. **Let us replace that silence with our voices.**

- that secrecy, whether it be professional, diplomatic or political exercised by services, lodges, associations, or sects, is the hiding place of truth. Tolerating it is to lie. **Let us replace the secrecy with openness.**

- that giving priority to titles is belittling the human values of respect, sharing, helping one another, and creativity. **Let us replace appearances with essence.**

- that fear is the death of conscience. Letting it kill us is to accept that someone else, who makes us afraid, controls our destiny. **Let us replace fear with willpower.**

- that in negating the sovereignty of the clients and in abusing our authority as doctors, we deny our own sovereignty and accept the authority of another over us. **Let us replace the power OVER with the power OF.**

To dominate is to accept to be dominated

THE TREATMENT: SOVEREIGNTY

Righting the system

The dispossession of the power of patients and doctors is achieved thanks to an all-powerful hoax. Namely, so-called "scientific" medicine. The two-step righting of the system consists of:

Step One: Re-establishing the sovereignty of the patient/client

From the very moment that patients take back their power and exercise their sovereignty and decisional power, they take back control of their money and health. They stop feeding the system of sickness, "scientific" medicine. For lack of food, the system dies. It disappears of its own accord. Without money, there is no longer a system. Can you imagine civil servants continuing to work without being paid?

No bloodshed. No revolution. But rather a change of power achieved quietly and calmly. Noblesse oblige!

This first step is **fundamental** and has never been done. All sorts of beautiful projects in the past failed because the first step was omitted. Only someone who is sovereign can exercise his power without being dominated and exploited. As soon as patients exercise their sovereignty as clients and employers, the authorities disappear. Both they and their established system. There is no longer any reason for them to exist.

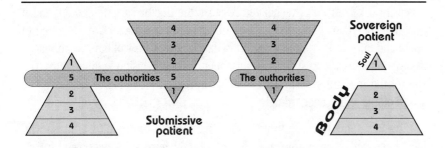

Step Two: Forming a patient/doctor partnership

Plugging the breach between patient and doctor, a breach which has allowed the authorities to infiltrate between the two. This means that doctors must also become aware of the illusion of "scientific" medicine and see it for what it really is. In addition, they must recognize the true sovereign of the medical system, the all-powerful patients, and put their skills at their service, their clients, their employers.

This second step is achieved automatically, once the first step is concluded. Because people who are equal always understand each other and get along. As nobody is trying to dominate the other. A win-win partnership is born.

STOPPING the social hierarchy

Based on inequality and inequity, the social hierarchy is man-made. It is a creation of human beings designed to exploit human beings. It is a creation of the privileged to maintain their privileges. They take for themselves the usurped rights of individuals and parcel them out. Some to the next less-privileged along the chain who, in turn, part some on to others who are even less-privileged. And so on and so on. That is how the hierarchy is created.

This authority exists only because we believe in it. It is nothing more than an illusion. What authority do we have over someone who does not wish to obey? None. We can always beat them, even kill them. But they will only obey if they decide to. We have only the authority that others wish to give us. Let us stop playing this game of power OVER others and apply ourselves to acquiring the power OF.

As patients, let us put our foot down!

Let us regain our rightful place in the social hierarchy. If we have lost it, and we have for centuries, it is because we ourselves have let it be taken from us. We have believed that others could heal us better than ourselves. That they were better equipped to make decisions for us than we were ourselves. That they were more competent than us, etc.

Medicine is first and foremost an affair of the heart. Who better than we to decide that which suits us best? In any case, it is our health and it is we who will live the results of our choice. Better that we make that choice ourselves. If we accept to have our child vaccinated because the doctor says we should, and if our child becomes paralyzed as a result, it is not the doctor who is going to come and take care of him or her every day. It is we who will have to do that. If we are going to have to suffer the consequences of a decision, let it be ours. The soul of the medical system, the essence, the reason for being, is us. Let us be aware of this and act accordingly.

Authority is for those who believe in it

We are going to run into resistance, particularly on the part of those who have been sitting on the thrones that we should have been occupying for all these years. We should always remember that the last thing the privileged are going to give up are their privileges. They will feel very threatened and will try to intimidate us and make us afraid. We should only listen to what our heart tells us. We will not go wrong. Let us begin by practicing it today. Let us no longer give our doctor the title "Doctor". Let us address him or her as we would address someone who is at our service. Mr. or Mrs. XYZ. Or even by their first name. Whatever we think best. And stop letting ourselves be called patients. We are clients of a counselor whose services we have retained and whom we pay from our own pocket. If we act in such a manner, we will be recognized accordingly. Doctors are not imbeciles. When they see that they are losing clients, they will adjust. It is we the clients, therefore, who must take the initiative and educate our doctors. If they are too stubborn and thick headed, go ahead and see another who is more open-minded.

IN THE SAME WAY THAT CHILDREN
EDUCATE THEIR PARENTS
WHEN THEY ARE GROWING UP,
CLIENTS EDUCATE THEIR DOCTORS.
IT IS THE NORMAL BALANCE OF NATURE.

Doctors, come back down to earth!

Ever since we began studying medicine, we have been taught to believe in our superiority over patients. Let us realize that if the authorities have given us power over others, it is their way of having power over us. We all lose in this game.

> **Off
> the Pedestal**
> Michael Greenberg

"Let us come down from our pedestal", urges our colleague Michael Greenberg in his marvelous book entitled *Off the Pedestal.*

As long as we maintain a hierarchal rift between we doctors, between ourselves and patients, between ourselves and hospital personnel, between ourselves and nurses, between ourselves and therapists, we will also be victims of this hierarchy. To play an authoritative role is to accept the authority of someone else over oneself.

We should remember that our patients can live without us. But we cannot live without them. Let us recognize that and let us tell it to them. Let us call them our employers. Let us use all our talent to help them. Even if we do not always agree with their opinions. Let us admit that their opinion is just as valid as ours. Have we never been wrong? After all, it is really a matter of their health, not ours.

Let us realize that we have only learned one sound of the bell toll in medicine, the *ding*. But a bell cannot peal without a *dong*. Yet we do not know about the *dong*. Let us recognize our limitations and learn more about alternatives to conventional treatments. Always with an open mind. In doing so, we will be able to offer a better range of solutions to our patients for their well-being.

Let us realize our helplessness in the face of the health system in which we operate. Let us share our fears and our concerns with patients. Let us realize that it is they who can free us from our golden prison. Only our lack of confidence and insecurity can make us act with authority. Let us not fear our patients. They are just as worried as we are. Let us make them our accomplices, our partners, rather than our adversaries. We will both be winners in the process.

Starting today, let us remove our masks and drop our facades. Let us become the uncomplicated people that we once were when we chose a profession of helping and devotion. Let us call ourselves by our names, without hiding behind the title. Let us also call our patients by their true name, our clients.

The authorities: an unnecessary evil

Like a broken record, we keep repeating that "Government is a necessary evil". And we believe it. We are so molded by the patriarchal system based on hierarchy and the leadership of the elite that we find it difficult to believe otherwise. We are afraid of disorder, abuse, anarchy.

Are we so irresponsible, so uncertain, and so incapable, that we must always have someone else judging us and directing our lives? And punishing us whenever they wish just like children? Even children do not need to be scolded or punished after a while. They begin to practice self-discipline. Why should it be any different with us adults?

Who are these people who purport to be our superiors? What gives them the right to call themselves authorities and appoint others to decide for us that which is good for us? Nobody. Absolutely nobody has the right to decide for us, nor judge us. **We should not let anyone usurp our fundamental right of managing our own lives and our freedom to choose. Nobody.** We allow people to usurp our power because we believe that we are unequal and that some people have more worth than others.

By putting our individual authority in the hands of others (power OVER) we have created the **governmental monstrosities** that we must deal with today, where technocrats who know only statistics and doctrines make all decisions regarding our health. We could not do worse than that. And they know it. In order to preserve their power, they cause us to argue between ourselves. They are not lacking in imagination!

And we dance to their tune without ever saying a word. While we are so busy arguing between ourselves, they continue to play with our health and our money. And we suffer in silence. And we foot the bill.

For our security

Security and protection are illusions

Can having our health money managed by a technocrat be any better than how we could do it ourselves? Who are they to tell us who, or what, is good and who, or what, is not? We can do that. Moreover, we pay for the service. There are good and bad professionals in every field, regardless of their degree of education. Sure, there must be a minimum of study. But it is not in school that we perfect our common sense. It is up to us to check out a professional's qualifications when we consult him or her, or even before. Then we can make up our own mind and trust our feelings and the comments of others who have used their services.

For our protection

The Medical Board (College of Physicians) is said to be for the **protection of the public**. Yet each time that the public needs its services, they run into a brick wall. Their file is passed from one committee to another, so that the issue is lost in paperwork. Or, it simply refuses to give out information. It is because of these failings that different groups have been created for patients with complaints. We have already seen this with vaccines. For those who have been sexually abused. There are independent groups which put out brochures and provide support committees. As for victims of plastic surgery, let's not even talk about that. The scandal of breast implants has proven that the authorities have known of the dangers of such implants for years. And yet they continued to authorize them.

Following the incompetence and ineffectiveness of the authorities to inform and protect us, one woman took the initiative. She created an agency providing information on esthetic surgery and those surgeons practicing it. It provides information on the types of surgery available, as well as the results, good or bad, of those surgeons who are practicing it. The data bank is based on the results of those operated on. Isn't that individual authority? It is a thousand times more effective than what the established authorities can, or would even want to offer us.

There are many examples that we can indeed do much better for our health and our wallet than the authorities!

Another trap that we should beware of, is that of **recuperation**. In France, for example, when it became impossible to forbid acupuncture and homeopathy because they were so popular with patients, the Board/College had no choice but to take them "under its wing". Since then, only doctors have the right to practice these disciplines. Taken over by the medical establishment.

We are making the same mistake when we want the authorities to recognize midwives. We should simply consult them and have them help us give birth at home. Period!

Employer-employee relationship

- The employer is the one who pays the salary of someone, either directly or indirectly. The patient is the employer.
- The employee is the one who is paid for doing a job. The doctor is the employee.

We are the employers of the medical and political authorities. Yet our employees make us call them "Doctor", "The Honourable", "Your Honor", "Your Majesty", and on and on...

In addition, they:

- ordain respect for their status
- decide without consulting us
- spend without counting
- steal our money against our will
- make laws to control us
- impose electronic systems to keep track of us
- train controllers to catch us
- pay judges to condemn us
- pay the police to punish us
- pay the soldiers to subdue us
- set their own salaries, pay increases and pensions
- and on and on it goes...

And all that with our money! We would never tolerate such behavior in our own company. But we do it in the two biggest companies. Health and society.

WHO IS AT THE SERVICE OF WHOM?

In medicine, as elsewhere, the employer is at the service of the employee. The system is upside down! It is because we have abdicated our individual rights, our sovereignty, that the authorities have taken it over.

I will never forget the face of a client who told me one day: "Doctor, I am sorry for taking up your time again, but I have another question to ask you." And I said to her: Madame, please continue to take up my time because, if you don't, I will find myself on welfare."She looked at me flabbergasted." After a few seconds of silence, she said: "But its true, you're right." To which I replied: "I know that it is true. Without you, I wouldn't have a job. It is you who is allowing me to make a living."

OFFICIALLY	IN PRACTICE
The employee is at the service of the employer	The employer is at the service of the employee

Let us resume our real roles

In practice, this means that the patient, the client, and the doctor resume their real respective role of employer and employee.

The client employer

The patients will take their rightful place, exercise their power, take back their **sovereignty**. This means that we as **clients**:

- Regain **control of our money**, never again doing business with intermediaries that are imposed upon us, private or public insurance companies.

- Pay cash without a receipt for services rendered.

- Stop the electronic **control** of information by the authorities. Stop using any form of health card. Keep our own data on our state of health, that is, keep our files with us.

- Stop signing any form of document relating to consenting to treatment, confirming the refusal of a treatment or of being vaccinated, etc. We alone are responsible for our health. Nobody else is.

- Ensure that all have **access to healthcare**, rich or poor. It is because of this lack that government has promised security for all and has established its control over health. Universality of healthcare, yes. But by government, no.

- Give donations at a local level, to those in need in the community. Never give or bequeath money to societies or other foundations for illnesses. These bodies support the establishment and are in the pay of the Medical Mafia.

- Change our own **sense of values**. Opt for sharing instead of possessing. For helping others instead of always thinking of ourselves.

- Take **responsibility for our own health** and for that of our communities. Also for the cost that this entails. And hold ourselves totally responsible for whatever happens to us.

- Completely **control** the medical system, medical schools, hospitals, etc. Organize medical conventions, and choose the subjects and the guests to be invited.

- Take remedies that are locally made. And made by people whom we know. Also keep a close eye on the intentions of the industry. Is it to provide a valid service or solely to **make a profit**?

A major reputable manufacturer of homeopathic products has just been *bought out by a giant car manufacturer...*

- Stop taking legal actions. Become informed before consulting. Make a clear decision.

- Realize that we have the cure in us and that we alone can cure ourselves.

- Do not ask the practitioner for a prognosis of the illness. How the illness evolves depends entirely upon us. We alone create its future.

- Demand that our doctors and therapists work together and that we make the final decision.
- Change practitioners if we are not well served. And explain why.
- Inform and educate our doctors and all medical personnel.
- Judge the quality of the office, reception, services, and let our feelings be known.
- Pay more for consultation than for treatment.
- Pay quickly and well, but never before having received a service.
- Pay for those who do not have, on a pro-rata basis, according to their means.
- Carefully screen and scrutinize any and all medical booklets talking about vaccination, medications, etc.
- Stop being duped by scaremongering in the media.
- Follow a normal pregnancy, without automatically resorting to a doctor, echography, tests. The experience of birth is a determining factor on the future psyche of the child. Giving birth at home with the help of a midwife is much less traumatizing.
- Take time to reflect and listen to our conscience.

The employee doctor

As **doctors**, we will reassume our rightful place and act as **advisers**. Come down from the pedestal and begin serving our clients. This means that we, doctors:

- No longer acts like gods or gurus, but as human beings equal in every way.
- Take the time needed to listen to, and examine our clients and make a clinical diagnosis.
- Charge more for the consultation than for the treatment or test.
- Reduce work hours and adjust lifestyles accordingly.
- Conduct ourselves in a professional manner, defend our opinions and stop practicing defensive medicine.
- Cancel our responsibility insurance and inform our clients that they alone are responsible.
- Establish a reasonable hourly rate and make the terms of payment easier, if necessary.
- Practice a medicine of health and shun all tests or medications that are not absolutely necessary.
- Respect the clients and treat them as we ourselves would wish to be treated.
- Use common sense and compassion.
- Stick to medicine and eliminate bureaucracy. Treat human beings and not files.
- Respect the decisions of the clients and work with them in their choice of therapy, even if it is not our own.

- Give the clients their diagnosis and hand over the files to them.

- Put the well-being of clients before all else.

- Never tolerate in silence any dangerous medicine being practiced by a colleague. No more "omerta" - code of silence.

- Do not make clients sign any document. There must be complete confidence. The clients must know that they alone are responsible for their health and the decisions they make.

- Become more open-minded and learn more about alternative medicines, as well as collaborate with therapists as equals, including midwives and healers.

- Learn more about medicine in books written by non-doctors so as to obtain information that is not controlled by the medical establishment.

- Never again accept a single favor, regardless of what it is, from the industry, particularly the pharmaceutical industry. Realize that even research that is subsidized by the industry in unacceptable. And that is not even talking about conventions, magazines, newspapers, perks, apprenticeships, trips, etc.

  To dominate is to accept to be dominated

- Stop feeling elitist. Remember that having authority over someone is to accept that someone has authority over us.

- Stop paying membership fees to the authorities, such as Collegio, Insurancio, and Associo. Stop belonging to associations and cancel subscriptions to medical magazines.

- Become involved in society, in neighborhood activities. Become part of the community.

- Drop prejudices. Clients are not "difficult", they are simply worried. They only need to be comforted and reassured.

As a rule, clients who at first seem to be difficult end up being the best *partners. I remember one who had come a long way to see me after having consulted several doctors, none of whom she was pleased with. As she entered my office, she took a notebook from her purse. It contained several pages of questions. I had already seen others with their list of questions. What I had never seen, however, was blank space immediately following the question, so that they could write down the answer. Right away, I knew why she had not gottten along with all the other doctors she had visited. I therefore decided to remain calm and not lose my patience. I replied to all the questions and waited while she wrote the answer to every one. That took some time, as you can imagine. But it was the best lesson of my life, because there seemed to be such a feeling of confidence and complicity between us, that all the subsequent treatments went as smooth as silk. To the satisfaction of us both. I learned that day how important it was to respect her concerns and wishes, and way of proceeding.*

- Welcome clients into a nice but not ostentatious office with an open reception area and friendly reception. Just imagine how you feel when you must knock on a little window, which is opened by someone who obviously wishes they were somewhere else, and which is then closed again. Just like in a prison.

- Visit clients at home. Spend some quality time with them. You will find answers to lots of their problems.

- Do not look upon clients as adversaries, but as partners.

- Establish a pool for those who do not have the means to pay. And encourage those who are better off to participate. Contribute your time.

- Say thank you, for the confidence that a client has placed in you.

- Write the medical file, simplified to the maximum, so that the client can read it.

- Never vaccinate again without putting the client fully in the picture. Do not prescribe medication of which you know nothing about.

Legal actions on trial

Lèse-majesté
=
to undermine
the majesty of
the sovereign

Legal actions are crimes of **lèse-majesté**. They deprive and constrain the rights of a person to their very core. Let me explain.

A sovereign is the person who holds the supreme power of decision. A sovereign is the supreme judge. Yet a legal action consists of asking someone else to assume that role of judge and decide in their place. Therefore, anyone who launches a legal action renounces their sovereign status, their fundamental right of being the supreme judge.

A legal action is **legalized violence**. The very same justice imposes a stronger right. It dispossesses individuals of their legitimate rights. It is based on a spirit of vengeance. It is revenge of the oppressed against the oppressor. Of the exploited against the exploiter. Of the dominated against the dominant. And the dominant, in the case of the patient-doctor relationship, is the doctor.

Hardly surprising that the patient seeks revenge against the violence of domination/exploitation by responding with violence. In this case, a legal action. Violence begets violence. Many doctors end up paying for the abuse of power by their entire profession and by the entire system. It is the revenge of frustrated patients. And not without reason.

A responsible
person is the
one who pays
the bill.

A trial is a **game of football** with two players on the field. The lawyers and a referee, the judge, who decides the fate of the patient by applying the rules of the game. Rules that have been established by the authorities and which have nothing to do with justice. In this macabre game, the patients are the indispensable object. The ball. Attacker and defender (the one who initiated the case and the one who is charged) are sometimes kicked in every direction so that the lawyers can earn their living playing the game. And it is we who pay for the admission fee.

Let us look at the **intention** behind a legal action. The goal of a legal action is to take money from someone by force. Against his or her wish. It is an act of legalized violence. It is resorting to an act of force to impose the will of someone on someone else. That of both the pursuer and the pursued. Rather than assume responsibility for whatever happens to us, we blast off against someone else. Making them the guilty party. And making them pay for our problems.

Yet, money never brings back health, and vengeance makes it worse. Therefore, the only way to be cured is to take responsibility (and that does not mean guilt) for our acts and for whatever happens to us. And to make an ally of our misfortunes. Lacking in wisdom, we learn by suffering. And in learning, we do not repeat the same mistakes. Let us at least afford ourselves the luxury of making new mistakes!

Who wins in a legal action?

Officially, the patient.
In practice, everybody, except the patient.

1. **Lawyers** who charge exorbitant professional fees, plus various costs related to specific areas of expertise, without counting the fact that they often take a percentage of the damages awarded by the court. When lawyers work strictly on such a percentage basis, for what is known as a contingency fee, they tend to make a deal with the opposite party's lawyer, whether the patient likes it or not. This, just before going into court, so as to avoid court costs which can be quite steep for them.

2. **Insurance companies** which make cases drag on for years so that the patient becomes worn out, discouraged, and gives up on a claim, or settles for very little. They also forbid doctors from doing anything that might bring their innocence into question. Failure to do so will mean that their insurance company will cancel their policies. There are many doctors who would have made fair reparations or paid reasonable damages, if they had not had lawyers and insurance companies come between them and their patients. When a lawyer opens a file, it is war. Just as doctors know only illness, lawyers know only litigation.

Better still, in order to keep the industry's mind at peace, as well as that of its accomplices, and allow them to continue their crimes without a worry in the world, the authorities have created "compensation funds" for automatic payment to future victims. Such is the case with vaccines.

Today, French and Canadian hemophiliacs, who became seropositive following a contaminated blood transfusion, are still impatiently waiting for their compensation. However, they have to realize that:

- They are not ill. Because seropositive does not mean AIDS. People who are seropositive are not ill. Unless they take AZT.

- In order to camouflage an enormous political scandal, they are being "paid off". They are protecting the giant financial interests of those engaged in the world-wide business of blood.

- They are in effect stealing from their fellow-citizens. I was even told by one French doctor that some of them, upon the advice of their lawyer, stopped receiving treatments that would otherwise have so improved their health that they would not be eligible for compensation.

Whenever they must pay, insurance companies readjust the premiums for responsibility insurance of doctors in light of damages they have had to pay out in the past, and those they expect to have to pay out in the future. To achieve this, they call upon the services of an actuary, whom they pay very generously to ensure that it will be just as profitable for them in the future as it was in the past. Unfortunately for us, they are very good at it. Doctors' insurance premiums go through the roof and, they in turn, pass the higher costs on to their patients. It is we, the patients, at the end of the line, who always end up paying. Even when the system is socialized.

We should remember that insurance companies are financial concerns created with the sole purpose of making profits and not rendering service. Once again, the patient is at the service of industry. And not industry at the service of the patient.

3. **Industry**, which makes us pay for its mistakes. When there are so many legal actions being taken out that the company could face bankruptcy, and the government was party to the hoax, the claimants are brought together in a "class action". They are led to believe that there is strength in numbers. Also that it will not cost them so much as they can share the legal fees. It is an illusion. It merely results in an agreement settlement for the victims paid by the government. In other words, it is we who pay, with our taxes, for the criminal mistakes made by manufacturers and their accomplices in authority. The silence of claimants is bought with their own money, that as taxpayers.

4. The **authorities**, medical and non-medical, who are delighted to see us arguing among ourselves as patients and doctors. Divide and conquer, such is their tool of domination. While we devote all our energy to fighting between ourselves, they do whatever they want. And in their own interests. Understandably, the authorities do nothing to stop this plague of legal actions in the field of medicine. On the contrary. They encourage it.

Who loses in a legal action?

Officially, the doctor.
In practice, all patients.

1. **The patients who win money** are not satisfied. They must spend months, and more often years, of waiting and frustration of all kinds before having their day in court. Here they will realize that it is only a pretext for a chess game. The outcome will be decided of its own accord. Whether it be right or wrong. If they do not get as far as the court, it is because lawyers, theirs and those of the insurance company, will have arrived at a settlement and will have strongly urged them to accept it. Money doesn't buy happiness. And victory does not rectify the mistakes.

I have been called as an expert witness on behalf of a patient who had been seriously injured by a medical treatment. The judicial process dragged on so long that, during this time, her husband left her and she had no means of supporting herself because she could no longer work. Nor had she yet received any compensation. I learned one day that she had committed suicide.

2. **The doctors being prosecuted** are, first and foremost, the big losers. Some live a nightmare which runs the full gamut. A feeling of defeat in the eyes of their peers. A feeling of being rejected by their patients. The fear of being reprimanded by the authorities, distrusted by their fellow-doctors, and being financially ruined by the lawyers. They are ashamed. They don't sleep. It also nourishes hatred against those they believe to be responsible for their misfortune. The lawyers. The patients. They then protect themselves by practicing defensive medicine. They will compensate by increasing their professional fees in proportion to the new insurance premiums that they will have to pay. And who do you think will pay this new bill?

3. **All patients are the big losers** in a legal action, on all fronts. Medical, financial, and moral.

   - On the medical level, they are served **defensive medicine**. They are treated like illnesses and not like sick people. The doctors no longer take any initiative for fear of being put on trial. They no longer treat patients, but files.

Because, on these files will focus the attention in a legal action. Since only that which is written counts, that's one rule of the legal game, doctors are going to fill out a lot of paper. And as only tests are credible, that's also a rule of the medical game, doctors are going to order a lot of tests. They do so simply because they are afraid of being accused of not having done enough. Tests substitute for comprehensive medical examinations. Silence for dialogue. Figures for common sense. Suspicion for complicity. That is what we, as patients, reap from our legal actions.

On the moral level, we act like victims. Incapable of taking charge of our life and how we live it. We become passive and obedient.

On the financial level, we **pay needlessly** for an **excessive number** of tests, visits, medications, hospitalizations that are not necessary. The big winners, at the end of the line, are the technological, pharmaceutical and other industries. It is therefore easy to understand why the authorities are in favor of maintaining legal actions.

Always remember that each time that we give our power to someone other than ourselves, we are victims, irrespective of whether we are the patient or the doctor.

So what are we to do?

First of all, take your own reciprocal responsibilities.
Then, create a client-doctor partnership.

Once the system is back on its feet, we can be assured that it will never be turned upside-down again. Let us replace the gap that exits between patient and doctor with a close relationship. Let us rid ourselves of the intermediaries who separate us.

THE CURE: SOLIDARITY

The only real
doctor is oneself

The cure, or healing, is the complete and definitive disappearance of the illness. To cure implies eliminating sickness **everywhere** and **forever:**
- the cause of the illness: submission, and replacing it with sovereignty;
- the tool of the illness: the hierarchal pyramid of domination and exploitation.

On account of our submission and the hierarchal pyramid of power of some OVER others, the medical system knew illness and disorder before becoming overturned completely.

We have therefore corrected these two problems:
- the submission of the patient has given way to sovereignty and the system has righted itself.
- the adversity that divided patient and doctor has given way to the partnership which unites them.

The patient-doctor partnership leads to the **crumbling of the hierarchal pyramid** of power of some OVER others. Indeed, this pyramid is like a house of cards. Take away a single card and it will collapse. Take away a single block of the pyramid and it will come toppling down. Take away a single level of domination, and the social hierarchy is no more. Whenever two people who are sovereign come into contact with one another, there is **fusion**, resulting in a sphere of power. That is **solidarity.**

Medical solidarity

Medical solidarity is the concrete result of the successive fusion of four groups of the medical system. It is accomplished in three steps.

1st step: the patient-doctor fusion

The sovereign patient initiates the first fusion, the patient-doctor partnership. The doctors cannot prevent it, whether they wish to or not.

2nd step: successive fusions

- **The doctor-services fusion**

  The doctors initiate the second fusion, the doctors-laboratories-hospitals-clinics-pharmacies partnership. In order to achieve this, the doctors will have first fused with therapists and healers. The doctors will also have come together among themselves. In other words, they will have eliminated their medical hierarchy of surgeons, specialists, and general practitioners.

- **The services-industry fusion**

  The services initiate the third fusion, the services-industry partnership. In order to achieve this, the services will have fused together by having replaced competition with collaboration. Industry follows their example.

3rd step: total fusion: medical solidarity

All the members of the medical system are working together, on an equal footing, for good health and the prosperity of all. Patients and those who look after their medical interests. It is the fusion of the bodies and the soul of the medical system. The medical system is definitively healed and cured.

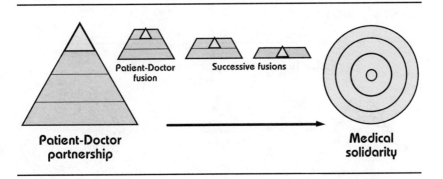

Universal solidarity

A partnership, whether it encompasses two or a thousand people, demands that each of the individuals involved recognize his or her own sovereignty and that of others. The power games of some OVER others is automatically eliminated. Everyone is equal. Domination, exploitation, possession, is finished.

NO PARTNERSHIP WITHOUT SOVEREIGNTY

One can see how the fusion of two blocks of the pyramid gives rise to the progressive fusion of other blocks of the pyramid and the collapse of the entire pyramid.

1. **Sovereign patients** recognize the sovereignty of their partners in life and of their children. The conjugal and family partnership replaces the power games between the parents and the parental authority over the children. The same type of relationships are established at work and at school. And the fusion grows.

2. **Sovereign doctors** recognize the sovereignty of patients, other doctors, specialists and general practitioners, therapists using alternative medicines, healers, nurses, and everyone involved in health. Partnerships multiply at all levels. Doctors recognize that everyone is equal to them, regardless of whether or not they have a diploma. All have the same importance and right to the same considerations. The same types of relationships are established in the home, with neighbors, and in the community. And the fusion grows.

3. **Universal solidarity** follows this progressive fusion. Ever more closely, all of the blocks of the pyramid fuse together and we find ourselves in another social structure altogether. A world where everyone is interdependent. One relying on the other. The health of each depends upon the health of all. And the health of all is reflected upon the health of each individual. It is the **power of one WITH others.**

We will then witness the coming together of all human beings within themselves, between each other, and with all the inhabitants of the planet. We are all fused together, with the Source of Universal Energy. **We are the Creative Universal Energy.**

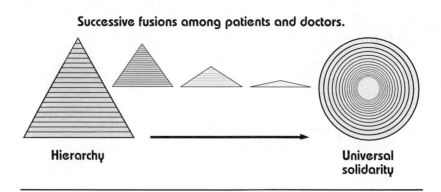

Successive fusions among patients and doctors.

Hierarchy   **Universal
                                  solidarity**

WHO IS GOING TO INITIATE THE REMEDYING OF THE SYSTEM?

We are kept people. We are waiting for government to provide the solution and bring about the necessary changes.

Yet we have seen that government is the very tool that was used to overturn the system in the first place and that it maintains it so today. **Government is never** going to make the changes that are required. Who is going to do it then? To determine which person is the best qualified to initiate the remedying of the medical system, let us look in a little more detail the function of each of the **CO-**llaborators in the Medical Mafia.

The 4 COs of the Mafia

If the Medical Mafia, or any other Mafia for that matter, remains in existence, it is because it can count on a whole hierarchal network, which serves it at all levels. From the top down, In order, there are **4 CO**llaborators of the Mafia.

COnspiracy

A conspiracy is a plot. That is to say a secret plan. If the element of secrecy is missing, there is no conspiracy. The medical conspiracy consists of reducing the patient and the doctor to a state of slavery at the service of the multinationals. It also strips everyone's control over their health by a single centralized world control, of which the representative is the World Health Organization. An organization that is itself largely infiltrated by pharmaceutical multinationals and world bankers.

COrruption

Corruption is the act of corrupting, causing someone to act contrary to their duty. For a bribe. It is the level of the establishment that **barters and trades in its soul for privileges**. A level that sells us out to the all-powerful to ensure their power. Money begets power. And power begets money. Multinationals set up and maintain governments which, in turn, wanting to remain in power, ensure the privileges of the multinationals. The philosophy is as old as time itself. "I scratch your back and you scratch mine". Medical corruption is to be found at the level of the medical establishment. To be precise, at the level of government (agencies responsible for health, health insurance, laws) and the bodies over which it has total control.

COmplicity

Complicity is participation in a crime. It is at the level of those charged with performing a task by the establishment. Sometimes consciously, sometimes unconsciously, they collaborate with the Mafia. Medical complicity is driven by those who work in the established health field, without always playing an influential role. They are agents of the system. And they include doctors. Either one is part of the solution, or one is part of the problem. They are part of the problem. These are the **"quiet accomplices"**.

COnsentment

Consentment is agreement. It is to accept that something has happened. Through silence and failure to act, it allows a crime to have taken place. It is the **omerta of the Mafia**. By saying nothing, they agree. Medical consentment is the patients who remain silent and who continue to obey a system which has totally abandoned them. They value security and protection to autonomy and responsibility. Slavery to freedom.

Let's take an example.

- I plot to rob all the banks in a major city and, as a result, take over control of the city. It is a secret plan and I do not tell anybody. That is **CONSPIRACY.**

- In order to carry out my plan, I retain the services of experts, professional bank robbers. I hire each of them to hit a specific bank. But I do not reveal my overall secret plan to anyone. I bribe them to make them commit a crime. That is **CORRUPTION**.

- To help them rob their allocated bank, each professional bank robber hires a driver who will drive the car and transport the money. The drivers are not aware that they will be driving a get-away car or carrying stolen money. They do their job without asking any questions. They are paid, without ever asking where the money came from. Sure, it all seems a little suspect. But it is best not to ask questions for fear of losing one's job. That's **COMPLICITY**.

- While all this is going on, two pedestrians happen by. They lean against a lampost to check out what is happening. There seems to be a lot of strange activity around the bank. But after a couple of minutes, they pass quietly on their way. They could have raised the alarm. And the robbery could probably have been averted. But they were afraid and preferred not to get involved. They kept quiet. They opted for omerta. By their silence, they consented to the robbery taking place. That is **CONSENTMENT**.

In this scenario, we note that the four levels of the Mafia, the **4 COs**, are essential for the success of the project. If just one of the four was missing, the robbery would have failed. The lesson to be learned is that we only have to concentrate our efforts on one of the four levels to stop the Medical Mafia. BUT WHICH ONE?

Do we think that we can change the mastermind's plan? No. Because we do not know who it is. It is a secret.

Do we think that we can change the minds of the professional bank robbers? No. Because they each have too much to lose. It is too lucrative a profession to just let it drop.

Do we think that we can change the accomplices? No. They also have too much to lose. They have a good job and are afraid that they will lose their share.

Do we think that we can change the idea of the passers-by? Yes. They have nothing to lose and everything to gain. All they have to do is whistle, cry out. Just let others know what is going on and everything will stop right there. After all, it is a conspiracy. A secret plan. Take away the secret and there is no conspiracy. The plan is dead.

So it is not at the level of the World Health Organization, nor the level of government, nor the level of doctors, that we must turn to, if we are going to see and realize the remedy of the system. It is at the level of the patient. The antidote to the Mafia is individual sovereignty. The CO of sovereignty is COnscience.

The COnscience

Conscience is the sovereign voice of your inner God/Goddess. It is through conscience that you will realize your sovereignty and power over the health system. Pharmaceutical multinationals control medicine, thanks to their enormous profits. But if you decide to no longer buy their medications, the industry will collapse, as will its power. That is true, real power.

You have the real power of the medical system. And it is you who will initiate the righting of the system. Because it is you who has the least to lose in re-establishing the health system. On the contrary, you have everything to gain.

The conscience is to the soul as the physical senses are to the body. It is the sense of the invisible, just as sight, hearing, smell, taste and touch are the senses of the visible. The conscience sees, hears, feels and manifests the inner reality. It reads thoughts, reads between the lines, understands body language, hears that which is not said, reveals to us the hidden face of things. **It is your contact with your inner divinity, your Light, your spirit**. It is to be found in the soul.

"One can only see well with the eyes of the heart."

St-Exupéry

PHYSICAL SENSES	CONSCIENCE
• senses the visible	• sees the invisible
• matter	• spiritual
• at the level of the body	• at the level of the soul
• informs us about appearance	• reveals to us the essence
• external information	• inner knowledge
• human	• divine
ILLUSION	**REALITY**

Conscience makes us see reality, that which is over and above the illusion of matter. It tells us whether spoken or written words are illusionary or real. It **enables us to distinguish** between truth and lies. To **go beyond** what a person is actually saying or writing in order to determine their intentions. It **dictates** what path we should take.

- The conscience can remain asleep and blind. Just like the average man or woman in the street. It allows the authorities to continue manipulating us. It is **quiet complicity**.

- The conscience may be awakened. But it lets fear take hold. And it is paralyzed. It is the conscience of **helpless submission**.

- The conscience can take the situation in hand and control its destiny. It is the conscience of **all-powerful sovereignty**.

Becoming conscious

Becoming conscious, becoming aware, triggers action. It is neither contemplative, nor passive. It means getting up from our seat in the audience of passive spectators and victims, and climbing up on to the stage. As an actor responsible for our destiny. This is achieved in three stages. The **3 Ps.**

- **P**erceiving reality
- **P**ermitting fear
- **P**osition taking

1. Perceiving reality

Our conscience makes contact with our inner voice. In order to do this, there has to be **silence**. Turn off the radio and the television. Get away from the noise for a little while each day. Spend some time alone. And listen. The truth will come. There will be light shed on reality, on that which doesn't please or suit us, on that which we want. And on our fears.

2. Permitting fear

Reality creates fear because it threatens our habit of illusion. This is why we do want to see it, or face up to it. Now that it has appeared, welcome it. And with it, the inevitable fear that accompanies it. Do not reject it. Identify it. Call it by its rightful name, what it is. And laugh at the fact that an illusion, like fear, can cause you to be upset. And sometimes even paralyze you.

Let's be honest. It is we who lie to ourselves. I cannot help but think of the policeman to whom I explained that parking tickets are illegitimate and who answered me: "I don't have any choice but to obey the law because I have a wife and children to support." To which I replied: "Have you ever asked them if they really want you to do this? That you sell your soul for them?" My question went unanswered. The policeman knew that I knew that he was afraid. He realized that he was lying to himself. How can one confront fear, if one pretends that it doesn't exist? Everyone has the right to be afraid. Even the policeman.

"Lying makes one ill."

Oscar Wilde

Once we recognize that we are afraid, we can then proceed to demystify and unmask it. Fear of what, of whom, why? Once that is established, we can then tackle it. Get right into it. Take our fear to the very extreme. **Stop dying OF fear. Instead, let our fear die**. Fear is an illusion which paralyzes the conscience. It is the master of emotions and thoughts. Wherever it hides, it is always fear that imprisons our love in its cage of hatred, jealousy, anger, resentment. And in the falseness of preconceived ideas.

3. Position taking

There are a thousand and one reasons for not taking a position. And they can all sound good. But isn't it crazy what tricks the mind can play on us? To make us lie to ourselves. When we say to ourselves: "I don't have a choice," what we are really doing is renouncing our human condition. As human beings we have a choice. An animal that is afraid, fights or takes flight. It has no choice. We can follow our instinct. We can also transcend it. This raises the questions:

- am I going to stay submissive to my fear, let it direct my life, and collaborate with the system?

Or...

- am I going to take charge of my life and object to the system?

WHO IS AT THE SERVICE OF WHOM?

> "One cannot serve God and Mammon (God-money)."
>
> Jesus Christ

"The right of every man is to listen to his conscience and his duty, and act according to that which it dictates."

This phrase of Albert Einstein reminds me of something that happened to my son in school. During a philosophy class, his teacher was expounding upon morality. She was explaining that one had to respect the laws and obey the rules established by the authorities. William, as a teenager was little inclined to obedience and with a mind of his own, began to discuss the validity of such laws. But without much success, his teacher having been trained in the school of obedience. When, suddenly, he had a brainwave. He asked his teacher what she thought, on a moral level, of Robin Hood. He of Sherwood Forest who robbed from the rich and gave to the poor. The teacher cut short the discussion, saying that she would answer him later. There's no point in explaining how frustrated my son felt. He told me how angry he was. Using my common sense, I told him that he had understood the difference between legality (laws) and legitimacy (conscience). But that the school authorities did not want to think about this. To make him feel a little better, I quoted this little phrase of Einstein, adding that both he and Einstein had understood the real difference.

VACCINATION
BE IT COMPULSORY
OR NOT

BY FORCE
IT IS RAPE

COLLABORATING
WITH IT IS DEADLY

Collaboration: collective complicity

Let us take vaccination for example. In order for vaccinations to be done, it takes the collaboration of all parties. Industrial, medical, political, education systems, and parents. That is the Mafia. It works thanks to the "omerta" of us all who participate in its realization, at whatever level. Some make the vaccine. Others sell it. Others announce it. Others impose it. Others inject it. Others lead our children to it. Like most people, we do it without ever questioning. Like the proverbial lemmings we jump into the sea. After all, the other lemmings are doing it. As we were taught, we repeat stereotypical phrases without even thinking twice:

- "For your protection", yet nobody asks to be protected unless they are afraid.
- "So as not to be responsible for the sick", as if anyone has ever been responsible for the health of others.
- "So as to avoid legal action", as if anyone could take legal action against us for being sick.
- "Because it is the policy of the institutions (school, hospital)", while it is we, patients, students, taxpayers, who are the bosses of everyone working in these very institutions. We have the sole right to make the laws and policies.
- "It is mandatory", while each individual has the right to determine what, if anything, is going to be put into his or her body.

Each step leading to collaboration with forced vaccination is just as deadly as that of a rapist stalking the streets. Both end up violating the body.

Non-collaboration: conscientious objection

The position of sovereign persons is entirely different. They obey their conscience, rather than that of the authorities. They are not stopped by the manipulation of fear and guilt. They rise above it. They make contact with their inner divinity, which reminds them that they are all-powerful and in perfect health, as they were created. They remember that vaccines are dangerous, ineffective, and that they disturb their inner ecology, in addition to draining their immune system. They decide to take the decision that THEY will decide to take. They decide to listen to their conscience and to do that which it tells them to do. It is as simple as that.

If their conscience objects to laws, rules or obligations **imposed by force and/or by the law**, they will declare themselves CONSCIENTIOUS OBJECTORS. They will proclaim that their only decision-making influence and judge are their conscience. They will act according to their SOUL AND CONSCIENCE. Nobody can object to this. It is such a strong sentiment that even the military authorities respect its "power". What can be more normal than refusing to kill?

Speaking and acting

Once we have made a decision as to whether to collaborate or not, proclaim it loudly. Taking a position is to speak and to act.

- SAY what camp we are in. Say it to ourselves, first of all. There is no good or bad. There is simply a choice between life and death. One must say it loudly so as not to be mistaken. Then say it to others so as to let them also become aware of their right and of their duty to become aware of it.

  To speak is to put an end to "omerta", the complicity of silence. All murderous acts are done with our collaboration, active or passive. Not speaking of what we see, is to be an accomplice. Not saying that vaccines are dangerous, for example, is being party to the usurpation of our rights. Journalists have never interviewed the many victims of vaccinations, simply because they are not around anymore. Everyone and anyone who has had problems resulting from vaccinations, needs to stand up and be counted.

- ACT in accordance with your choice. Never accept the unacceptable. Make sure that every act and step is in accordance with the choice you have made. Be true to yourself.

  Maintaining the status quo is to accept submission. Opting for a better world, is passing from submission to sovereignty, and choosing health/life. This passage is called transformation. It happens in our daily actions when we break with our old habits. And the rebirth of new ways of acting.

Say NO to the 3C's of submission

1. **No to confrontation**

   Let us stop playing the game of the enemy: divide and conquer. We are all sovereigns of divine essence, therefore equal. Let us realize that the authorities create scapegoats to deflect our anger. More often than not, they are the minorities, be they black, white, native American, women, the poor, the homeless, homosexuals, blue collar workers, etc. Let us realize that we live in a world of violence regardless of country. The direct result of the hierarchal domination of some OVER others.

   Let us take back our power OF, our inner power. And we will also see the divinity of all other living souls in the world. Make the book of Machaelle Small Wright our motto, "Act as if God/Goddess in each human being was important". In his marvelous book, which I recommend to everyone, Serge Mongeau teaches us: "Peace is not utopia". And peace can be learned. Always remember that: that which we do not like in others is always the mirror of that which we do not like in ourself.

2. **No to cards**

   Be wary of credit cards, automatic teller cards, health insurance cards, hospital cards, cards of any kind. Also cards for vaccinations and medications. They are used to track us down, code and classify us. They are the tool of *Big Brother*. They know everything we do. You believe that your medical file is confidential? Well, it sure isn't to civil servants and others like authorities! They have access to all the information it contains. We can live without cards. Pay cash and stay far away from computers, as long as they are controlled by the authorities.

What's more, let us put an end to running into debt, the tool of our slavery. To be in debt is to submit to the oppressor. Begin by lending money to your relatives and friends. The Mafia does it, why shouldn't you?

3. **No to consumerism**
Consumerism is a really bad habit. It is an addiction. Saying no to consumerism is really nothing more than that. It is being conscious of how one spends one's money. Buy only what you need. Support your local economy. Avoid chainstores, products from multinationals and imported products. Always basing one's purchases on the lowest price, is to act irresponsibly.

Let us not forget the golden rule of our economic survival: "Buy all that we make and make all that we buy." Marcia Noczik tells us how to do it in her book, **No Placc Like Home.**

> **No Place Like Home**
> Marcia Noczik

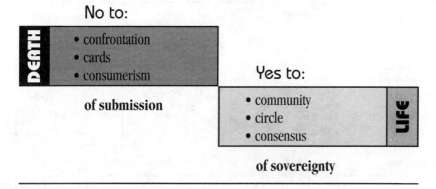

No to:

DEATH	• confrontation • cards • consumerism		LIFE
	of submission	Yes to: • community • circle • consensus	
		of sovereignty	

Say YES to the 3C's of sovereignty

1. **Yes to the community**
Let us realize that we, alone, can do nothing. We are interdependent. And nobody is going to save one's skin alone.

   EITHER WE WILL ALL BE RICH OR, WE WILL ALL BE POOR

The community is made up of sovereign people joining together. We are all equal, without exception. The community constitutes the basic unit.

2. **Yes to the circle**
No-one is worth more than the other. Wise people do not need diplomas in wisdom. We find them and we consult them. Everyone participates equally. Everyone's views count. No domination, no exploitation.

3. **Yes to consensus**
Decisions have to be taken unanimously. Decisions cannot be imposed by a simple majority. How do you feel when six people out of ten decide on a course of action while four others disagree strongly? And you are one of the four?

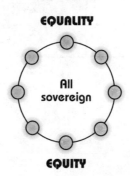

EQUALITY

All sovereign

EQUITY

Transformation of the conscience

	▽	△	◎
Level of consciousness	collective submission	individual sovereignty	universal solidarity
State of the system	over-turned boat	boat righted	unsinkable
Power	power OVER	power OF	power WITH
Authority (divinity)	external	inner	fusion with Source
State of health	sickness-aging-death	health-youth-life	unlimited health
Reply to the fundamental question	soul at the service of the body	body at the service of the soul	life eternal body and soul fused with the Source
Kingdom	material	spiritual	divine
Energy	procreator	co-creator	creative
Structure	division	duality	unity
Vibrations	heavy	light	subtle
Medium of evolution	matter	spirit	pure spirit
Organization	established (dis)order	natural order	Cosmic Universal Law
Relations	attack	defense	peace
Attitude	suffering	stand up	transcend
Action	spectator	actor	direct

Transformation of the conscience

A transformation is much more than a mere change. It is much more than improving a caterpillar by giving it legs. It is transforming its very essence. To become a butterfly. Transformation is an "initiation". That is to say, a **passage**, from one state to another. The caterpillar must die in order for the butterfly to be born.

THE FIRST TRANSFORMATION of the conscience is available to us all. It consists of the death of submission and the birth of sovereignty. The death of those emotions and thoughts that imprison us, coming to know freedom at last. To act like a sovereign is to let oneself be guided by one's conscience and not let external powers, or forces, dictate the path we take. Our inner power is to be found in our soul, as is our life program and our conscience. We have within us the tools of our sovereignty.

LIFE

DEATH

LIFE

THE SECOND TRANSFORMATION of the conscience will follow the first. It consists of the demise of the hierarchy and the birth of equality and equity. It is the advent of true **universal solidarity**. The transformation of the conscience is something that has to be worked at every day. Every moment. In all circumstances. In all one's thoughts, words, emotions, and actions. It is simple. In the words of my daughter Valerie, one only has to:

"Without being re-born you will not enter into the Kingdom of Heaven."

Jesus Christ

TURN SHIT INTO GOLD

Every moment of our life can be heaven or hell. One only has to bring it forth from the darkness of the material world for it to shine in the light of the spirit.

Conscience and health go hand in hand. The level of our conscience determines the state of our health. The higher level of conscience, the higher the vibrations of our bodies. And the better our health. The transformation of our conscience is definitely the key to good health.

SHIT	GOLD
sickness/death	health/life
war against the external enemy	peace with the friend within
sad thoughts	happy thoughts
separation from god	oneness with God/Goddess
suffering	joy
victim	responsible
glass ½ empty	glass ½ full
dying of fear	the death of fear
caterpillar	butterfly
submission	sovereignty
power OVER	power OF
external god	God/Goddess within
darkness	light
HELL	**HEAVEN**

DAVID AND GOLIATH

The patient is all-sovereign and all-powerful

I can already hear you saying that this is impossible. That the government is all-powerful and that we can do nothing against such a behemoth. That they have all the powers. And that they can crush us whenever they wish. But we should know that nothing is impossible. Let us remember the story of David and Goliath. Don't we feel like David right now? Like a little poor shepherd boy in the shadow of a giant who is armed to the teeth, who is threatening us with slavery. If that is the case, let us remember how the story really went. And let us take inspiration from it. It was certainly told so that it would serve us one day. Well, that day is long over due.

The story

There was once an army which wanted to beat a people into submission. To conquer them. To avoid an all-out battle and the deaths of many, the attackers proposed a duel, between only two men. One from each of their camps. Their man was already chosen. He was a terrifying giant of a man, wearing heavy armor and armed to the teeth. He was called Goliath.

He was so fiercesome a sight that nobody in the other camp wanted to challenge him. All seemed lost when, suddenly, a young boy stepped forward. Dressed like a shepherd boy, he carried only a sling-shot. He had come to defend his people against the aggressor.

The duel began. But David had seen a small, vulnerable spot where Goliath was unprotected. He picked up a stone and, whirling the sling-shot, he aimed for that very spot. He hit his target and Goliath crashed to the ground.

Little David had defeated the colossus, Goliath, to the astonishment of all. He had saved his people from slavery.

IF IT WORKED FOR DAVID, IT CAN WORK FOR US

The example

Let us look closely at how the fight to the death between David and Goliath went down. A blow-by-blow analysis, if you will, so that we can perhaps draw lessons from it to assist us in our fight. We can identify five major points:

1. David decided not to be overcome by fear.
2. He identified the enemy.
3. He found the weak spot in the armor.
4. He used an extremely simple tool, or weapon.
5. He won.

We only have to do the same to get out of the crushing and threatening situation in which we find ourselves right now. By applying these same five points to our current situation. Let us:

1. Take the decision to no longer let fear cripple us and take control of our life. Fear paralyses the conscience. One cannot see anything, hear anything, or feel anything. One is like a deer in the glare of a car's headlights. One is a slave to whoever, or whatever, is creating that fear. It is a decision that has to be taken. If we do not, it is opting for the status quo, submission and slavery.

2. Identify the real enemy that is hidden behind what appears to be a giant. Look beyond appearances and become conscious of the very essence of the aggressor of our freedom. The apparent giant is the medical, governmental and administrative authorities. It is the big machine that makes us afraid with its laws, its police, its prisons, its army.

   But it is important to see that this facade is created by the privileged in order to maintain their privileges. The real enemies are the world financiers. It is they who pull the strings of their giant puppets.

3. Find the weak spot which makes the enemy vulnerable. Remember, the armor is only made of paper, bank notes that we willingly hand over every day of the week. The enemy's power rests in our money that we give it.

4. Use a very simple tool, or weapon, to vanquish the enemy. All we have to do is to stop giving them our money. It is the ***VELCRO SOLUTION***, whereby we put *Velcro* on all our pockets in order to stop supporting the enemy and its armies. We will then be rich and free, as opposed to being poor and enslaved.

5. Visualise the victory. Have faith. Imagine a better future and create it. Nothing less than a paradise for sovereigns! We will come to know health and wealth.

In practice

I can already hear your shouting. "It is not all that serious. I'm used to it." Let us look at the three most common causes for reluctance:

- the authorities
- human nature
- utopia

The authorities

"The authorities will never let us do it!" That's true. The last thing they are going to let go of are their privileges. How could it be any other way? They are going to hang on to them any way they can. Don't wait for their blessing. We are going to be threatened, they are going to try to scare us, and we are going to be attacked by all their arsenal of manipulation. The authorities cannot control us without our consent. The only true power that exits is our inner power. Nobody can take that away from us.

David is daring, but not suicidal. He will never fight using the weapons of his enemy. What are they? The law. You probably know or have heard of someone who spent a lot of time, energy and money trying to fight "city hall". Never forget that that is their strength. The authorities make and change the laws as they wish, to suit their needs.

For example: whenever a strike lasts too long for their liking, the authorities simply pass back to work legislation. This is what happens to a right which our ancestors fought for decades to aquire. In addition, the authorities conduct trials with public funds, our money. We pay our costs and theirs. The same reasoning applies to force and weapons. Never, never, never resort to violence. The authorities are past masters at making us fight between ourselves. It is their favorite tactic. Don't fall into the trap. Always remember who the real enemy is.

Civil war is the supreme art of "divide and conquer."

David had a sense of community and knew that in unity there is strength. The first thing to do, therefore, is to band together in our respective neighborhoods in order to take charge of our health. The objective is simple and attainable. To reduce surgical procedures as well as the taking of tests and medications of which the large majority are useless and damaging. Let us treat social problems with social solutions and not with pills and surgery. Illnesses are of a social origin and do not cost a lot to resolve.

For example: There is a grandmother, who takes 15 pills a day and who, as a result, is a zombie. Then there is Richard, who is out of work and who spends much of his time in front of the television. He could visit with her every day. Help her to get out, write letters for her to her friends, make telephone calls to her children. And he would be able to talk about a thousand and one things, to someone who has the time to listen. Both of them would feel useful. Both of them would feel proud and that they have a friend. Everyone would be richer. And, the grandmother will probably need far less pills.

We can multiply this example thousands of times. Let us have confidence in our imagination.

Abundance for all

- **The United States**. Because the system is non-socialized, it is still possible to take back one's power and regain control over one's money. As it is employers who pay the major portion of health insurance, why not reach an agreement with them. One which will see both parties come out winners. For example: we can propose to our employers that they pay us, the employees, the amount that they paid in insurance premiums last year. We will then be entirely responsible for our own health. If the costs exceed last year's expenditures, we will assume the difference. If the costs are less, we will share the savings with our employer. We do not need the government to do that. There are always solutions when one wants to find them.

- **France and Canada**. Here the freedom of health has been lost. Money is deducted directly at source, without consent. One can always plead that this is unconstitutional, but then one has to fight using their legal weapons. Why not ask the government to send everyone an itemized bill for their individual health expenditures for the previous year. People can then organize themselves into "health" groups and after a year of operating as such, do the same itemization. Calculate how much each member of the group saved in sickness insurance by practicing a medicine of health for a year. Then the group claims the savings back from the government. While I don't expect anyone will receive a reimbursement in the next day's mail, this money is owed. It becomes a debt that the government owes the individual groups. Maybe the groups could withhold a portion of their taxes to help the government pay this debt. It may sound far-fetched at first, but think about it.

Whatever the formula, we will soon realize how profitable our actions can be when we regain control over our money and health.

Multinationals control us by their riches. But these riches come from us. If we stop buying their pills, they will not sell them. If they do not sell them, they will no longer make enormous profits. If they are no longer rich, they can no longer buy the medical system and corrupt those who direct it. And so on and so on. **The *Velcro* solution is all that and more!**

Human nature

" Human nature is corrupt and corruption always rears its ugly head." "One will never change human nature."

No, this is not human nature. It is our perception. Human nature is corruptible, but is not corrupt in its very essence. We are intelligent beings, endowed with freedom of choice. Our intelligence determines whether we are corrupt or not. The choice is not predetermined. We make it every day, every moment. The opinion that we have of others is the mirror of that which we have of ourselves. When we say "people are like this or like that", substitute the words, "I am like this or like that."

Darkness can do nothing against the light

Think of ten people who are closest to you and try and find an example of corruption. Perhaps, sometimes, one in ten. Is 10% of the population really a significant figure? No. So why do we think this way? It is because, for centuries, the authorities have nourished this illusion, to cause us to squabble and bicker between ourselves. For centuries, we have repeated the same old refrains, such as: "man is man's own worst enemy", without ever realizing that we are capable of transcending our instincts. By debasing human nature, we act accordingly. Elevate it, and we will each conduct ourselves like a sovereign God/Goddess. It is up to us to choose. We are the creators of our future.

Utopia

"It is utopian!" Yes, it is utopian. So much the better. And I add a phrase that really captures my true thoughts:

"Utopia or death"
René Dumont

One that is similar to that on New Hampshire's license plates:

"LIVE FREE OR DIE"

I have chosen life! And you? I invite you to join me. As we approach the end of a turbulent century, we seem to be rushing towards our own extermination and global totalitarianism. Both of which are the result of our materialistic choices pushed to the extreme. It is not a question of continuing to make little changes. Either we transform our old scheme of references, or we die. Now you may want to reply to the question:

IS THE SPIRIT AT THE SERVICE OF MATTER
OR
IS MATTER AT THE SERVICE OF THE SPIRIT?

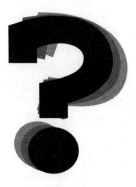

Who is at the service of whom?

SOCIALIZED MEDICINE FOR AMERICANS?

"Socialized Medicine is to Americans what a Bicycle is to a Fish"

This was the title of a conference that I gave in Chicago at the beginning of 1990. Today, here, I repeat the same thing with more certainty than ever.

The facts: there are two problems

What is not working in the health system in the United States? It is simply **too expensive** and **not accessible to all**. That is it in a nutshell.

1. TOO EXPENSIVE

All sickness systems are expensive. Only health is economical. That is why all existing systems, socialized or not, and regardless of the country, cost so much that they are pushing all countries towards ruin. In addition, they do not satisfy anyone, except of course those who profit from the practice of a medicine of sickness, which does not cure or heal.

SICKNESS ALWAYS COSTS TOO MUCH

Ever since the Flexner Report was implemented in 1910, **scientific medicine** was put in place by force and alternative medicines have been eliminated. Based on the concept of **war against an external enemy**, scientific medicine uses a sophisticated, technological arsenal, a jargon all of its own, and robotic technocrats to wage its war.

WAR ALWAYS COSTS TOO MUCH

Let us bear in mind that even words are very misleading:
- health system means a system of sickness
- health insurance means sickness insurance: it pays sickness,
  it ensures sickness, not health
- A Health Security Card means Sickness Guarantee Card
- A National Health Board means National Board for Administration
  of Sickness.

2. NOT ACCESSIBLE TO ALL

The system of sickness that we have is not accessible to all. Not only because of the system itself, but **because of poverty, the fruit of social injustice**. It is this social injustice that we must correct first and foremost, not the system of sickness.

In countries where socialized medicine is already in place, there is also a parallel pay-as-you-go type of medicine for the rich. Those who can afford to pay to get first class service, while the poor have to be content with second best. Some have to wait for hours, and even months, for certain services. It is by cutting more and more guaranteed services, that is to say by reducing the services themselves and the public's accessibility to them, that the government has succeeded in holding down constantly soaring costs.

And although the rich do have to pay even more to maintain the former level of services, many are no longer available to the poor. The poor are again losers. As for doctors, they also lose out. The cuts force them to work even harder and faster. While the only winner, industry, continues to amass astronomical profits!

"Competition is a sin."
John D. Rockefeller

Why has our system of health assumed such prohibitive costs? Who, if not the international financiers and scientific medicine that support it, profit from such sums of money? Remember one thing:

"In politics, nothing happens by chance."
President F. D. Roosevelt

Let us ask ourselves why the authorities have waited so long to propose socialized medicine to us, if it is the best solution. In France, it has existed since 1950. In Canada, since 1970.

And if it is not the best solution, why do the authorities wish to impose it upon us when other countries, convinced that it has been a disaster, have been trying to get out of it for years?

" In politics, nothing happens by chance."

Either it is good and it should have been done earlier. Or it is bad and should never be done at all. Do we really want to put our health totally in the hands of government?

- Either our government works for us. Just look at how it has shown its incompetence in the small part that is under its control. *Medicare* and *Medicaid* . One can only shudder at the prospect of what would happen if it controlled the entire system of sickness.

- Or our government works for the world financiers. Then it has been an accomplice to the financial exploitation of our health. Do we want to give total power to those who betray us?

Could it be that all has been set up by the authorities for many years? With the intention of causing us to give up our freedom of health? All the ingredients are there to make us so frustrated with the present system that even a socialized system with its centralized bureaucratic control would be welcomed as a deliverance. After all, nothing could be worse. Or could it?

"In politics, nothing happens by chance."

The myths: and they are many

Myth

Socialized medicine will be administered at the least cost by one standard insurance, as opposed to being administered by thousands of different private, independent insurance companies.

Reality

Passing from 1,500 independent insurance companies to one governmental controller, is to pass from competition to a monopoly. A monopoly exists when all control is in the hands of one entity. Yet one of the sickness programs proposed stipulates that:

> *"Health benefits would be established and viewed periodically*
> *by a national health board appointed by the President."*

In practice, this means that the control of recognized services and their costs is in the hands of a single committee. One person names the members of the committee, and that same person controls the health of each and every American. A monopoly couldn't do better.

Yesterday's freedom	Today's control	Tomorrow's monopoly
No managers / 1 2 3 4	Managers	Managers
250,000,000 controllers	1,500 controllers	1 controller

Whoever says monopoly says exclusive control over prices and services. The patient who must deal with a monopoly is at its total mercy. It is passing from a multiple form of power to a single form of power. It is giving a blank cheque, for life, to someone without any restriction whatsoever and forever. It is paying in advance, without any recourse, for a service, the content of which we do not know. Nor are we sure that it is needed. Would we ever walk into a store and pay in advance, without knowing what we were going to buy?

Moreover, payment is obligatory. And the amount to pay is determined by a committee, whether we are sick or not. If we all opt for health and not sickness, we must still continue paying for sickness.

In reality, we have need of neither government, nor insurance companies, to administer our health and our money. We are going to do it ourselves. We are going to insure ourselves between ourselves. It will be much more effective and much less costly. And we will all be in better health. A service for all, by all, tailor-made for us.

SOCIALIZED MEDICINE IS A BICYCLE FOR A FISH

Myth

The system of sickness in the United States is the worst, as we have heard repeatedly.

Reality

The system of sickness in the United States is the best, because one can still get out of it. It is much easier to get out of the system of sickness in the United States because there is still a choice between giving, or not giving, one's money to insurance companies. One can lay down conditions when considering a policy and refuse it, if it doesn't live up to expectations.

Under a State-controlled system, however, the government has exclusive control over the practice of medicine and its costs. It decides which medicine it will recognize and which it will reimburse.

Sick or not, it automatically takes money from our pockets. It can regularly increase the amount without our consent and use it as it sees fit. **One cannot get out of it**, even if one wants to take charge of one's own health.

SOCIALIZED MEDICINE IS A BICYCLE FOR A FISH

Myth

Only government can ensure universal care.

Reality

Government is not a guarantee of social justice. Every person has a right to health. Right! But not under the terms defined by world financiers and their health branch, the World Health Organization .

We are really lacking in imagination if we really believe that only a Big Brother government can guarantee universal care.

It really is having a low opinion of ourselves, we who are sovereign patients. We know that from now on we will rediscover health and wealth. We are all in a perfect position to guarantee ourselves universal care at an unbeatable cost.

SOCIALIZED MEDICINE IS A BICYCLE FOR A FISH

Myth

By controlling medicine, government will finally be able to pass laws that are necessary to ensure the greater freedom of therapeutic choices.

Reality

Why hasn't it done that already? In the socialized medical systems, as well as in the United States, alternative medicines are ridiculed and forbidden. The smothering of such medicines is very subtle in France, less subtle in Canada, and not at all subtle in the United States. But let's not kid ourselves. Freedom of therapeutic choice does not exist in western countries. Everywhere, the practice of medicine is strongly controlled by governmental organizations, in the pay of industry. Hopefully the Constitution, which was written to guarantee the rights of citizens against the abuse of power by the authorities, will see to the guarantee of freedom of choice in terms of medicine and health.

While the Ninth Amendment guarantees all freedom to all individuals but, as it does not specify the medical field in particular, it will have to wait for a decision of the Supreme Court to this effect. And the Supreme Court will rely on the recommendations of experts, recognized by the authorities!

SOCIALIZED MEDICINE IS A BICYCLE FOR A FISH

Myth

Without socialized medicine, and if the current growth rate of expenditures continues, we will be bankrupt.

Reality

Countries that already have a system of socialized medicine are already at this point. Therefore, let us ask ourselves why, for many years, the big names in high finance have been in favour of the health system? Either through their participation on commissions, or through the information that is put out which is financed by them. Why do they push socialized medicine? Have they all suddenly become philanthropists? It is certainly not their usual custom. Since when have they been concerned about people's well-being? Let us put ourselves in their shoes for a few minutes and try to understand their interest in socialized medicine.

- First of all, there is a mass of clientele not yet fully exploited. The 38 million Americans who are unable to buy insurance. It is a big untapped market that sickness insurance will deliver to them on a silver platter. And the people will pick up the cost.

- Secondly, it stabilizes their consumer sickness markets for their multinationals. One client, the government, is much easier, particularly when one controls it. At the same time, they are going to get rid of giant competitors, private insurance companies, once and for all.

- And lastly, they are financiers, don't forget. As bankers, their speciality is to make and provide money with interest. Sickness insurance will bring in enormous expenditures which the supplementary taxes will not be able to make up. The bankers will see to that.

SOCIALIZED MEDICINE IS A BICYCLE FOR A FISH

Myth

Socialized medicine is the only and inevitable solution to the problems of our current system of sickness.

Reality

Having to choose between the current medical system and socialized medicine is like having to choose between being punched in the face or kicked in the behind. Both hurt.

What a lack of imagination! Why take for granted that the solution must be painful, unpleasant, and also costly? The right reply, because there always is one, is that if the authorities really wanted to find a good solution, they would propose to us several scenarios, from which the ideal solution would emerge.

So while, on the one hand, Canadians are convinced that their health system is the best in the world, on the other, Americans are convinced that theirs is the worst in the world.

As we have confidence in the authorities, we believe these myths and all conclude that "one must adopt a socialized system similar to that of Canada". Financiers have been preparing this scenario for years. The brainwashing has born fruit and we are now convinced that it is the only solution. A big mistake!

There is no excuse for ignorance, particularly when one is so close to that supposed role model country. We have had the opportunity to watch their health system evolve over the past 25 years. Let us go and see the bankrupt Canadian system for ourselves. Then we will be able to draw our own conclusions, rather than letting the authorities do it for us.

We have the luxury of coming up with something new, the first of its kind. It is more stimulating for the imagination and much more enriching for evolution.

SOCIALIZED MEDICINE IS A BICYCLE FOR A FISH

Myth

Socialized medicine is a means of smoothing out the differences between rich and poor and of ensuring a fair allocation and distribution of money.

Reality

It is not a question of the distribution of money. But rather the REdistribution of money that has already been unequally distributed from the beginning.

All forms of taxes, allowances, compensations, sickness insurance, unemployment insurance, grants, forms of financial assistance, scholarships, pensions, or guaranteed incomes, are the means of REdistribution of money. Not by the rich to the poor. But by the less poor to the poorest of all. From those who still have jobs to those who no longer have one. It is always the same monetary mass that is earned by the work of some that is shared out with others.

Real distribution is done well before REdistribution. It was done at the precise moment that the rich took possession of our riches - natural, industrial and services - the heritage of all the population. They seized and exploited them for their own profit, which they did not distribute at all. The only part that they did relinquish was in the form of salaries. And then only because they didn't have any choice. Even there, they are now moving their companies to under-developed countries in the Third World in order to pay as little as possible and replace workers with robots.

"Power is always charged with the impulse to eliminate human nature, the human variable, from the equation. Dictators do it by terror or by inculcation of blind faith; the military do it by discipline; and the industrial masters think they can do it by automation."

E. Hoffer

Real distribution is therefore done between owners, who reap the profits of the exploitation of our riches and from workers, who reap the salary of their work. It is ONLY this salary that is REdistributed.

SOCIALIZED MEDICINE IS A BICYCLE FOR A FISH

Myth

Raising taxes to allow millions of people to be taken care of and easing pressure on companies, which have to carry the burden of health insurance, is commendable.

Reality

It is a fancy way of skirting around the Constitution. All increases in taxes that are not consented to are anti-constitutional. Let us also not forget that in 1913, Congress granted private banks the right to make their own money. And it is because of this decision that we are stuck with the so-called debt that has cost us so much in interest charges.

SOCIALIZED MEDICINE IS A BICYCLE FOR A FISH

Myth

Socialized medicine is an evolution over capitalist medicine. It denotes a concern for others and a sense of sharing.

Reality

Capitalism, socialism, communism, liberalism. All are identical regimes and forms of government. Only the label varies. All of these regimes have one common denominator. Control of the majority by the minority. Power in the hands of a privileged clique who pass the laws necessary to maintain their privileges.

Socializing health is repatriating it entirely, in both financial and practical terms, into the hands of a few. It is therefore much easier to control than when it is in the hands of many. It is true that we made a mistake somewhere along the line. We have allowed social injustice and the resultant poverty. Let us recognize that. And correct that.

SOCIALIZED MEDICINE IS A BICYCLE FOR A FISH

Myth

Ensuring all of security in the case of sickness, is to ensure everyone of freedom.

Reality

Freedom and security are two antagonists. The more one has of one, the less one has of the other. And vice versa.

We have already sunken into materialism and individualism. But from there to sink into blindly giving up our power into the hands of the government is a very big step.

The Fathers of the Constitution is are surely turning over in their graves. They remember well that the more oppressive legality there is, the less freedom there is. But what will they do when they learn that there are those who would trade freedom for security in opting for socialized medicine? With the total loss of freedom of our health and our right to freedom of choice. Both essential to the growth and happiness of every individual.

SELF-MANAGED MEDICINE IS TO AMERICANS
WHAT WATER IS TO FISH

CONCLUSION
Choice of a health system

The rule is the same for every system. Whether it is a question of a medical system, or of our own individual system. Their state of health is a reflection of what we do with our power. The power to think, feel, act. The choice is in our hands. We can give up our power or we can exercise it. Because we have the power to choose between:

Staying in the nightmare of yesterday: Sickness-aging-death

If we give up our power to the authorities, the law, fear, peer pressure, etc., we **submit** ourselves to the domination of others over us. We do not take decisions which are in harmony with our essence. With that which we really are. We live in a world of appearance, of illusion, of the material. Our soul is at the service of our body. The traveller is at the service of the vehicle. Without control over our destiny, it drives us towards sickness, aging, and death.

POWER OVER = EXTERIOR POWER = SUBMISSION = SICKNESS

Or, moving forward: Health-youth-life

If we keep our inner power and exercise it, we will conduct ourselves as **sovereign individuals**, all-powerful and responsible. We will take decisions that are in harmony with our essence, with that which we really are. We live in a world of reality, of spirit. Our body is at the service of our soul. The vehicle is at the service of the traveller. In controlling our destiny, we direct it voluntarily towards health, youth, and life.

POWER OF = INNER POWER = SOVEREIGNTY = HEALTH

To accomplish the dream of tomorrow: Unlimited health

If we fusion our inner powers of individual sovereigns, one with one another, we become **interdependent** and in **solidarity**, one with the other and with the Universe. We are Creative Universal Energy, unlimited in time and space. We are in perfect control of our vibratory frequency, of our state of health. We are then on the road to unlimited health, of eternal life.

POWER WITH = FUSIONED POWER = SOLIDARITY = UNLIMITED HEALTH

Each time you think, feel, or act, ask yourself:

DO I WANT TO EVOLVE TOWARDS SICKNESS OR TOWARDS HEALTH?

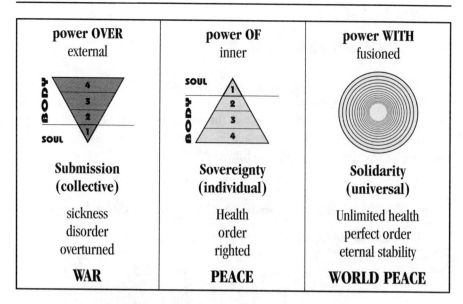

power OVER external	power OF inner	power WITH fusioned
Submission (collective)	Sovereignty (individual)	Solidarity (universal)
sickness disorder overturned	Health order righted	Unlimited health perfect order eternal stability
WAR	PEACE	WORLD PEACE

NO SOLIDARITY WITHOUT SOVEREIGNTY

The only real

SOVEREIGNTY

is

INDIVIDUAL

because it is

DIVINE

Generalization of all the systems

We now know how the medical system works:

- How it came to be overturned and capsized: Submission.
- How to right it: Sovereignty.
- How to navigate it, and sail it to infinity: Solidarity.

As a result, we also know how the smallest to the biggest systems work. For any system, whatever the field, the nightmare and the solutions are the same everywhere.

The system has always turned over and is upside down.

The soul of the system is always at the service of the body of the system.

The big beneficiaries are always the same, under different names, according to the system.

Their goal is always the same: to control, dominate, and exploit.

Their means are always the same: divide and conquer.

Their work is always done in the same way: in secrecy.

Their intermediary is always the same: government.

Their lie is democracy, in which all but they believe.

Regardless of the field, however deep it has sunk, it is possible to get out of it and find the light. To do this, we must open the door that we have been locked behind for years. That of submission. We all have the master key without which no door can be opened. We only have to use it. That is...

INDIVIDUAL SOVEREIGNTY!

Field	Submission	Sovereignty	Solidarity
HEALTH	submissive patient	sovereign client	unlimited health for all
ECONOMY	submissive taxpayer/ consumer	sovereign client	unlimited riches for all
JUSTICE	submissive citizen	sovereign individual	unlimited justice for all
COMMUNICATIONS	submissive parent/child	sovereign client	unlimited knowledge for all
EDUCATION	submissive parent/child	sovereign child	unlimited creativity for all

Yesterday's nightmare: **collective submission**

The patient is at the service of the system of sickness

They are exploited by doctors
health service providers
pharmaceutical and technological industries

which make people sick and keep them dependent to enrich themselves.

The taxpayer/consumer is at the service of the monetary system

They are exploited by accountants & book-keepers
economists
bankers

who impoverish, enslave and continue to dominate and exploit.

The citizen is at the service of the judicial system.

They are exploited by lawyers
courts, law enforcement
legislators

who usurp legitimate rights, make the laws, impose them by force in order to maintain their privileges.

The reader/listener is at the service of the propaganda system.

They are exploited by the media
experts
opinion leaders

who manipulate.

The child/parent is at the service of the system of obedience.

They are exploited by teachers
universities and intellectuals
think tanks

who teach obedience to the authorities and established order.

Reality of today
Individual sovereignty

Dream of tomorrow
Universal solidarity

Epilogue

I REMEMBER...
BUT I HAD FORGOTTEN

There was once a horse with wings
Who incarnated creativity and all
spiritual things.
Light as the wind, free as the air
He moved with the speed of a
lightning flare.
Because he knew no boundary
He was called ETERNITY

But one day man organized society.
Established his order and made his law.
He forbade the horse so mighty
From running and flying as before.
The winged horse let his wings wither
To let him gallop joyfully hither and
thither.
But the horse saw his legs become
shorter.
Working for man, he now had
responsibilities.
The horse saw his hair change to wool
For the profit of the authorities.

THE WINGED HORSE
HAD BECOME A SHEEP

A sheep that was black
Which had accepted to trade
Its wool for security
That was man-made.
Soon it was to see
That the shearing was increased
And the food was decreased.
In great disarray
He went to see Mother Nature not
far away

Who reminded the sheep:
"Remember that
In times gone by
You were a winged horse

Soaring high
Independent and resolute.
That nobody could refute"

The black sheep replied:

"I remember"

The black sheep returned to the
meadow, where
It explained to the sheep
assembled there:

"Enough of being fed
Just for the wool on our backs.
It is time to organize
And stop being hacks"

The black sheep left to wander alone
Throughout the world far from home.
Its wool to offer to all who would buy.
It walked so well
That its legs grew high and longer.
It jumped so far
That its wings grew back even stronger.

THE SHEEP THAT WAS BLACK
HAD TURNED BACK
INTO A WINGED HORSE

Poets rediscovered their inspiration

And the sheep their insubmission

FAREWELL SECURITY
LONG LIVE LIBERTY!

Suggested reading list

PROLOGUE

Δ   Bach, Richard: **Jonathan Livingston Seagull** (U.S.A., 1970)

Δ   Brennan, Barbara Ann: **Hands of Light - a guide to healing through the human energy field** (U.S.A., 1987) (ISBN 0-553-34539-7)
Bantam New Age

Δ   Brennan, Barbara Ann: **Light Emerging - the journey of personal healing** (U.S.A., 1993)(ISBN 0-553-35456-6)
Bantam New Age

Δ   Fontaine, Dr Janine: **La médecine des chacras** (France, 1993) (ISBN 2-221-07499-8)
Éditions Robert Laffont

Δ   Fontaine, Dr Janine: **La médecine du corps énergétique - une révolution thérapeutique** (France, 1983) (ISBN 2-221-01161-9)
Éditions Robert Laffont

Δ   Fontaine, Dr Janine: **Nos trois corps et les trois mondes** (France, 1986) (ISBN 2-221-04961-6)
Éditions Robert Laffont

Δ   Pedneault, Hélène: **Pour en finir avec l'excellence** (Québec, 1992) (ISBN 2-89052-494-9)
Éditions du Boréal, Diffusions Dimédia, Québec

PROBLEM

Δ   Chèvrefils, Dr Paul-Émile: **Le leurre médical** (Québec, 1982)
a/s Richard Chèvrefils, 430 rue Jarry Est, Montréal H2P 1V3 Tél.: (514) 385-5115

Δ   Enrenreich, Barbara and English, Deirdre: **Witches, Midwives and Nurses - A history of women healers** (U.S.A., 1973)(ISBN 0-912670-13-4)
The Feminist Press/Talman Company, 150 Fifth Avenue, New York, NY 10011

Δ   Flexner, Abraham: **Medical Education in the United States and Canada** (U.S.A., 1910) (ISBN 0-405-03952-2)
The Carnegie Foundation, 589 Fifth Avenue, New York, NY, U.S.A.

Δ   Illich, Ivan: **Medical Nemesis** (U.S.A., 1975) (ISBN 2-02-005661-5)
Bantam

Δ   Kramer, Heinrich and Sprenger, James: **Malleus Maleficarum**
Dover Publications, 180 Varick Street, New York, NY 10014, U.S.A.)

△ Lexchin, Dr. Joel: **The Real Pushers - a critical analysis of the Canadian drug industry** (Canada, 1984) (ISBN 0-919573-27-4)
New Star Books Ltd., 2504 York Avenue, Vancouver, British Columbia V6K 1E3

△ Michelet, Jules: **La sorcière** (France, 1966)
Éditions Flammarion

△ Nechas, Eileen and Foley, Denise: **Unequal Treatment - what you don't know about how women are treated by the medical community**
(U.S.A., 1994) (ISBN 0-671-79186-9)
Simon and Shuster, 1230 Avenue of the Americas, New York, NY 10020, U.S.A.

△ Payer, Lynn: **Disease-Mongers - how doctors, drug companies and insurers are making you feel sick** (U.S.A., 1992) (ISBN 0-471-00737-4)
John Wilet and Sons, 605 Third Avenue, New York, NY 10158-0012, U.S.A.

△ World Health Organization/United Nations: **Primary Health Care - the Declaration of Alma-Ata** (International, 1978) (ISBN 92-4-154128-8)
WHO/UNICEF/UN

SOLUTION

△ Bird, Christopher et Tomkins, P.: **The Secret Life of Plants**
(U.S.A., 1973) (ISBN 2-266-03757-9)

△ Chopra, Dr. Deepak: **Ageless Body, Timeless Mind - the quantum alternative to growing old** (U.S.A., 1993) (ISBN 0-517-59257-6)
Harmony Books/Crown Publishers/Random House, 201 East 50th Street, New York, NY 10022

△ Chopra, Dr. Deepak: **Quantum Healing - exploring the frontiers of mind/body medicine** (U.S.A., 1989) (ISBN 0-553-34869-8)
Bantam Books

△ Cousins, Norman: **Head First - the biology of hope**
(U.S.A., 1989) (ISBN 0-525-24805-6) E.P. Dutton, New York, NY, U.S.A.

△ DeMarco, Dr. Carolyn: **Take Charge of Your Body - women's health advisor**
(Canada, 1994) (ISBN 0-9694766-1-2)
Well Woman Press, P.O. Box 66, Winlaw, British Columbia V0G 2J0

△ Gerber, Dr. Richard: **Vibrational Medicine - new choices for healing ourselves** (U.S.A., 1988) (ISBN 0-939680-46-7)
Bear and Company, Santa Fe, NM 87504 - 2860, U.S.A.

△ Jampolsky, Dr. Gerald: **Love Is Letting Go of Fear**
(U.S.A., 1979) (ISBN 0-553-24518-X)
Bantam Books

△ Kroeger, Reverend Hanna: **The Seven Spiritual Causes of Ill Health**
(U.S.A., 1988)
Chapel of Miracles, Boulder, Colorado, U.S.A.

Δ   Lebrun, Maguy: **Médecins du ciel, médecins de la terre**
    (France, 1987) (ISBN 2-221-05247-1)
    Éditions Robert Laffont

Δ   Majnoni d'Intignano, Béatrice: **Santé, mon cher souci** (France, 1989)
    Éditions Jean-Claude Lattès/Économica

Δ   Marquier, Annie: **Le pouvoir de choisir - un paradigme pour l'émergence
    d'une nouvelle conscience** (Québec)
    Éditions Universelles du Verseau, C.P. 1074, Knowlton, Québec J0E 1V0

Δ   Martin, Dr Frédéric: **La foi sans croyance - l'éclosion de l'instinct
    de guérir** (France, 1992) (ISBN 2-86681-038-4)
    Les Deux Océans, 19 rue du Val-de-Grâce, 75005 Paris, France

Δ   Mongeau, Dr Serge: **Adieu médecine, bonjour santé**
    (Québec, 1982) (ISBN 2-89037-133-6)
    Québec/Amérique, 450 rue Sherbrooke Est, bur. 801, Montréal H2L 1J8
    Tél.: (514) 288-2371

Δ   Mongeau, Dr Serge: **Pour une nouvelle médecine**
    (Québec, 1986) (ISBN 2-89037-306-1)
    Québec/Amérique, 450 rue Sherbrooke Est, bureau 390, Montréal H2L 1J8
    Tél.: (514) 288-2371

Δ   Pekkanen, John: **M.D. - doctors talk about themselves**
    (U.S.A., 1988) (ISBN 0-440-50028-1)
    Bantam Doubleday Dell Publishing Group, 666 Fifth Ave., New York, NY 10103

Δ   Rosner, Iulius: **Requiem pour la S.É.C.U. - peut-on être mieux soigné?**
    (France, 1990) (ISBN 2-87671-074-9)
    Éditions Frison-Roche, 18 rue Dauphine, 75006 Paris, France

Δ   Roy, Jean-Hugues: **Profession: médecin** (Québec, 1993) (ISBN 2-89052-585-6)
    Les Éditions du Boréal/Diffusion Dimédia

Δ   Rubik, Beverly: **The Inter-relationship Between Mind and Matter**
    (U.S.A., 1992) (ISBN 0-9633272-0-8)
    Center for Frontier Sciences, Temple University, Ritter Hall 003-00, Philadelphia
    PA 19122, U.S.A.

Δ   Shapiro, Dr. Martin: **Getting Doctored - critical reflections on becoming
    a physician** (Canada, 1978) (ISBN 0-919946-09-7)
    Between the Lines, 229 College Street, Toronto, Ontario M5T 1R4

Δ   Siegel, Dr Bernie: **Love, Medicine and Miracles - lessons learned about
    selfhealing from a surgeon's experience with exceptional patients**
    (U.S.A., 1986) (ISBN 0-06-091406-8) Perennial Library, Harper & Row,
    10 East 53rd Street, New York, NY 10022, U.S.A.

Δ Weed, Susun S.: **Healing Wise - a wise woman herbal**
(U.S.A., 1989)(ISBN 0-9614620-2-7)
Ash Tree Publishing, P.O. Box 64, Woodstock, NY 12498, U.S.A.,
Tél./fax: (914) 246-8081

Δ Weston, Walter: **Praywell - a holistic guide to health and renewal** (U.S.A.
1994)Transitions Press, P.O. Box 618, Wadsworth, OH 44281, U.S.A.
Tél.: (800) 886-5735

OBSTACLE

Δ Bonhomme, Dr Jean: **Diafoirissimo, ou la déraison médicale**
(France, 1991) (ISBN 2-7103-0471-6)
La table ronde, 9 rue Huysmans, Paris 6e, France

Δ Dem, Marc: **Fric santé - le scandale** (France, 1992) (ISBN 2-268-01370-7)
Éditions du Rocher, 28, rue Comte-Flix-Gastaldi, Monaco/Jean-Paul Bertrand,
Éditeur, France

Δ Koch, Egmont R.: **Sang rouge, sang noir - chronique d'un scandale médical**
(France, 1990) (ISBN 2-87671-280-6)
Éditions Frison-Roche, 18 rue Dauphine, 75006 Paris, France

Δ Mullins, Eustace: **Murder by Injection - the story of the medical
conspiracy against America** (U.S.A., 1988)
The National Council for Medical Research, P.O. Box 1105, Staunton
VA 24401 or order from America West Publishers, P.O. Box 2208, Carson City
NV 89702, U.S.A.

Δ Mendelsohn, Dr. John: **Confessions of a Medical Heretic - tells you how
to guard yourself against the harmful impact upon your life of doctors,
drugs and hospitals** (U.S.A., 1979) (ISBN 0-446-30627-4)
Warner Books Inc., 666 Fifth Ave., New York, NY 10103, U.S.A.

Δ Ruesch, Hans: **Naked Empress - the great medical fraud**
(Switzerland, 1982) (ISBN 3-905280-07-8)
CIVIS Publications, Tal-Str. 40 CH-7250 Kloisters, Switzerland or: Fondazione
Hans Ruesch, Via Motta 51, CH-6900 Massagno-Lugano, Switzerland

Δ Walker, Martin: **Dirty Medicine - science, big business and the assault
on natural health care** (UK, 1993)
Slingshot Publications, B.M. Box 8314, London, England WC1N 3XX

Δ Wohl, Dr. Stanley: **The Medical Industrial Complex**
(U.S.A., 1984) (ISBN 0-517-55351-1)
Harmony Books, Crown Publishers, One Park Avenue, New York, NY 10016, U.S.A.

Δ Bell, Robert: **Impure Science - fraud, compromises and political
influence in scientific research** (U.S.A., 1992) (ISBN 0-471-52913-3)
John Wiley & Sons, 605 Third Avenue, New York, NY 10158-0012, U.S.A.

Δ Larivée, Serge: **La science au-dessus de tout soupçon**
(Québec, 1993) (ISBN 2-89415-118-7)
Éditions du Méridien

Δ Davesnes, Jean-Clair: **L'agriculture assassinée**
(France, 1992) (ISBN 2-85190-072-2)
Éditions de Chiré, 86190 Chiré-en-Montreuil, France

Δ Kneen, Brewster: **From Land to Mouth - understanding the food system**
(Canada, 1989) (ISBN 1-55021-050-5)
N.C. Press Ltd, Box 452, Station A, Toronto, Ontario, Canada

Δ Gritz, Colonel James "Bo":**Called to Serve** (U.S.A., 1991) (ISBN 0-916095-38-4)
Lazarus Publishing Company, Box 472 HCR-31, Sandy Valley, Nevada 89019, U.S.A.

Δ Marion, Pierre: **Le pouvoir sans visage - le complexe militaro-industriel**
(France, 1990) (ISBN 2-253-05541-7)
Calmann-Lévy/Le livre de poche

Δ Executive Intelligence Review: **Dope, Inc. - the book that drove
Kissinger crazy** (U.S.A., 1992) (ISBN 0-943235-02-2)
Ben Franklin Booksellers, 107 South King Street, Leesburg, VA 22075, U.S.A.
Fax:(703) 777-8287 - Tél. à Montréal: (514) 385-5495

Δ Coquidé, Patrick: **La médecine scandale** (France, 1993) (ISBN 2-08-066749-1)
Flammarion

Vaccines

Δ Berthoud, Dr Françoise: **Vacciner nos enfants ? - le point de vue de trois
médecins** (Suisse1985) (ISBN 2-88058-027-7)
Éditions Soleil, 32, avenue Petit-Senn, CH 1225, Chêne-Bourg, Suisse

Δ Buttram, Dr. Harold E. and Hoffman, John Chriss: **Vaccination and Immune
Malfunction** (U.S.A., 1982) (ISBN 0-916285-36-7)
The Humanitarian Publishing Company, P.O. Box 193, Richlandtown,
PA 18955-0193, tél.: 1 (800) 282-0677, U.S.A.

Δ Buttram, Dr. Harold: **The Dangers of Immunization** (U.S.A., 1979)
The Humanitarian Publishing Company, P.O. Box 193, Richlandtown,
PA 18955-0193, tél.: 1 (800) 282-0677, U.S.A.

Δ Buttram, Dr. Harold: **Vaccination and Immune Malfunction** (U.S.A., 1979)
The Humanitarian Publishing Company, P.O. Box 193, Richlandtown
PA 18955-0193, tél.: 1 (800) 282-0677, U.S.A.

Δ Chaitow, Leon: **Vaccination and Immunization: Dangers, Delusions
and Alternatives - what every patient should know**
(England, 1987) (ISBN 0-85207-191-4)
The C.W. Davis Company Ltd, 1 Church Path, Saffron Walden, Essex, CB10 1JP
England, tél.: 011-44-799-521909, fax: 011-44-799-513462

Δ   Chèvrefils, Dr Paul-Émile: **Les vaccins, racket et poison?** (Québec, 1965)
    a/s Richard Chèvrefils, 430 rue Jarry Est, Montréal H2P 1V3 Tél.: (514) 385-5115

Δ   Coulter, Harris and Loe Fischer, Barbara: **DPT, A Shot in the Dark - why the
    P in DPT vaccination may be hazardous to your child's health**
    (U.S.A., 1991) (ISBN 0-89529-463-X)
    Avery Publishing Group, Garden City Park, New York, U.S.A.

Δ   Coulter, Harris L.: **Vaccination, Social Violence and Criminality - the medical
    assault on the American brain** (U.S.A., 1990) (ISBN 1-55643-084-1)
    North Atlantic Books, 2800 Woolsey, Berkeley, CA, U.S.A., tél.: (510)644-2116
    Fax (510) 652-4336

Δ   Couzigou, Dr Yves: **Phobie des microbes et manie vaccinale** (France)
    Vie et action, 388 bd Joseph-Ricord, 06140 Vence, France ou: Ligue Nationale
    pour la Liberté des Vaccinations, B.P. No 9, 75430 Paris Cedex 09, France

Δ   Delarue, Fernand et Simone: **La rançon des vaccinations**
    (France) (ISBN 2-903009-05-8)
    Ligue Nationale pour la Liberté des Vaccinations
    B.P. No 9, 75430 Paris Cedex 09, France

Δ   Delarue, Fernand: **L'intoxication vaccinale**
    (France, 1977) (ISBN 2-02-004732-2)
    Seuil, 27 rue Jacob, Paris, France ou: Ligue Nationale pour la Liberté des
    Vaccinations, B.P. No 9, 75430 Paris Cedex 09, France

Δ   Delarue, Simone: **Les vaccinations dans la vie quotidienne
    (guide pratique)** (France)
    Ligue Nationale pour la Liberté des Vaccinations, B.P. No 9, 75430
    Paris Cedex 09, France

Δ   Delarue, Simone: **Vaccination/protection: mythe ou réalité ?**
    (France) (ISBN 2-903009-06-6)
    Ligue Nationale pour la Liberté des Vaccinations, B.P. No 9, 75430
    Paris Cedex 09, France

Δ   Ferru, Dr Marcel: **La faillite du B.C.G. - témoignages d'hier
    et d'aujourd'hui** (France, 1977) (ISBN 2-9500150-1-8)
    Ferru B.P.7, 95210 St-Gratien, France ou: Ligue Nationale pour la Liberté
    des Vaccinations, B.P. No 9, 75430 Paris Cedex 09, France

Δ   Grigoraki, Pr.: **Tuberculose et vaccin B.C.G.** (France)
    Ligue Nationale pour la Liberté des Vaccinations, B.P. No 9, 75430
    Paris Cedex 09, France

Δ   Honorof, Ida and McBean, E.: **Vaccination the Silent Killer** (U.S.A.)
    Honor Publications, P.O. Box 346, Cutten, CA 95534, U.S.A.

Δ   James, Walene: **Immunization - the reality behind the myth** (U.S.A.)
    Bergin and Garvey, 1 Madison Avenue, New York, NY, U.S.A.

△ Ligue Nationale pour la Liberté des Vaccinations, **Dossiers détaillés sur plusieurs aspects de la vaccination, notamment la Guerre Biologique** B.P. No 9, 75430 Paris Cedex 09, France - distributeur au Canada: Biosfaire, 312 Ontario Est, Montréal H2X 1H6 tél.: (514) 985-2467, fax (514) 843-8288

△ Mendelsohn, Dr Robert S.: **Raising Healthy Children... in spite of your doctor** (U.S.A., 1984) (ISBN 2-88058-039-0)

△ Neustaedter, Randall: **The Immunization Decision - a guide for parents** (U.S.A., 1990) (ISBN 1-55643-071-X) North Atlantic Books, 2800 Woolsey Street, Berkeley, CA 94705, U.S.A. or: Homeopathic Educational Services, 2124 Kittredge Street, Berkeley, CA 94704, U.S.A.

△ O'Mara, Peggy - editor: **Vaccination, the Rest of the Story - a selection of articles, letters and resources 1979-1992** (U.S.A., 1992) (ISBN 0-914257-10-2) Mothering, P.O. Box 1690, Santa Fe, NM 87504, U.S.A.

△ Randolph Society: **How to Legally Avoid Unwanted Immunizations of all Kinds** (U.S.A.) Humanitarian Publishing Co., R.D. 3, Clymer Rd., Quakertown, PA 18951

video

△ **Bad Vaccines** (U.S.A., 1994) NBC / NOW

△ **Consequences of Mass Vaccination** (U.S.A., 1979) CBS / 60 Minutes, 4/11/79

article

△ Horowitz, Carol, **Immunizations and Informed Consent** (U.S.A., 1994) Mothering, Winter 1993

AIDS

△ Bingham, Bill: **Biohazard, the Silent Threat - from biomedical research and the creation of AIDS** (England)
National Anti-Vivisection Society, 261 Goldmark Road, London South West
Great Britain, U.K.

△ Callen, Michael: **Surviving AIDS** (U.S.A., 1990)
Harper Collins, New York

△ Cantwell, Dr. Alan: **AIDS and the Doctors of Death - an inquiry into the origin of the AIDS epidemic** (U.S.A., 1988) (ISBN 0-917211-25-1)
Aries Rising Press, P.O. Box 29532, Los Angeles, CA 90029, U.S.A.
Tél.: (213) 462-6458

△ Cantwell, Dr. Alan: **AIDS: the Mystery and the Solution - the new epidemic of acquired immune deficiency syndrome**
(U.S.A., 1983) (ISBN 0-917211-08-1)
Aries Rising Press, P.O. Box 29532, Los Angeles, CA 90029, U.S.A.
Tél.: (213) 462-6458

△ Cantwell, Dr. Alan: **Queer Blood - the secret AIDS genocide plot**
(U.S.A., 1993) (ISBN 0-917211-26-X)
Aries Rising Press, P.O. Box 29532, Los Angeles, CA 90029, U.S.A.
Tél.: (213) 462-6458

△ Chirimuuta, R. and R.: **AIDS, Africa and Racism** (England, 1987)
Bretby House, Stafford, England

△ Coulter, Harris: **AIDS and Syphilis: the hidden link**
(U.S.A., 1987) (ISBN 1-55643-021-3)
North Atlantic Books

△ Girard, Rollande: **SIDA: tristes chimères** (France)
Éditions Grasset, Paris, France

△ Harris, Robert and Paxman, Jeremy: **A Higher Form of Killing** (1982)

△ Konotey, Ahuler: **What is AIDS?** (England, 1989)
Tetich-A Domeno Co, Watford, England

△ Krupey, G.J.: **Secret and Suppressed, chapter: AIDS: Act of God or the Pentagon?** (U.S.A., 1993)
Feral House, P.O. Box 3466, Portland, OR 97208, U.S.A.

△ Lauritsen, John P.: **Poison by Prescription - the AZT story**
(U.S.A., 1990) (ISBN 0-943742-06-4)
ASKLEPIOS/Pagan Press, 26 St-Mark's Place, New York, NY 10003, U.S.A.

Δ   Markoff Asistent, Niro: **Why I Survive AIDS - one woman's inspiring recovery - and the techniques she uses to help others** (U.S.A., 1991) (ISBN 0-671-68352-7) Fireside Books/Simon & Schuster, 1230 6th Ave., New York, Ny 10020

Δ   Nussbaum, Bruce: **Good Intentions - how Big Business and the Medical Establishment are corrupting the fight against AIDS, Alzheimer's, cancer and more** (U.S.A., 1990) (ISBN 0-14-01-6000-0) Penguin Books, 10 Alcorn Avenue, Suite 300, Toronto, Ontario M4V 3B2

Δ   Segal, Jacob: **New Directions in AIDS Therapy** (Sweden, 1991)

Δ   Shilts, Randy: **And The Band Played On - politics, people and the AIDS epidemic** (U.S.A., 1987) (ISBN 0-14-01-1369-X) Penguin Group

Δ   Snead, Dr. Eva Lee: **Some Call It AIDS, I Call It Murder - the connection between cancer, AIDS, immunizations and genocide - vol. I and II** (U.S.A., 1992) (ISBN 0-922356-59-9) AUM Publications, 126 E. Ridgewood Court, Suite 2700, San Antonio TX 78212, U.S.A., tél.: (512) 826-6613

Δ   Strecker, Dr. Robert: **Bio-Attack** (U.S.A.) Video: The Strecker Group, 1216 Wilshire Blvd., Los Angeles, CA 90017, U.S.A.

video

Δ   Strecker, Dr. Robert: **The Strecker Memorandum** (U.S.A., 1986) U.S.A.: Aries Rising Press, P.O. Box 29532, Los Angeles, CA 90029, U.S.A.

articles

Δ   Root-Bernstein, Robert, **Rethinking AIDS. Frontier Perspectives,** (Fall 1992) p.11.

Δ   Seale, John: **Scientific articles in the Journal of the Royal Society of Medicine:** 1988: 81: 537-39; 1989: 82: 519-22. Also in Nature 1988: 335: p. 391.

bulletin

Δ   **Rethinking AIDS** -James Trabulse, publisher, 2040 Polk Street, suite 321 San Francisco, CA 94109.

organisation

Δ   **H.I.V. Connection ?** -1072 Folsom Street, suite 321, San Francisco, CA 94103.

Cancer

Δ Bird, Christopher: **The persecution and Trial of Gaston Naessens - the true story of the efforts to suppress an alternative treatment for cancer, AIDS and other immunologically based diseases** (U.S.A., 1991) (ISBN 0-915811-30-8) H.J. Kramer, P.O. Box 1082, Tiburon, CA 94920

Δ Cantwell, Dr. Alan: **The Cancer Microbe** (U.S.A., 1990) (ISBN 0-917211--01-4) Aries Rising Press, P.O. Box 29532, Los Angeles, CA 90029, U.S.A. Tél.: (213) 462-6458

Δ Lynes, Barry: **The Cancer Cure That Worked - fifty years of suppression** (U.S.A., 1987) (ISBN 0-919951-30-9) Marcus Books, P.O. Books 327, Queensville, Ontario L0G 1R0 Canada Tél.: (416) 478-2201

Δ MacNaney, Christopher: **Cancer - new connections** (U.K.) People's Research Centre, Alston, Cumbria, U.K., CA9 3RF Tél. (0434) 381842

Δ McGrady, Patrick: **Cancer Scandal -the politics and policies of failure** (U.S.A.) Video/American Science Writers Association, U.S.A.

Δ Moss, Dr. Ralph W.: **Cancer Therapy - the independent consumer's guide to non-toxic treatment and prevention** (U.S.A., 1992) (ISBN 1-881025-06-3) Equinox Press/Movable Type, 331 West 57th Street, Suite 268, New York NY 10019, tél.: (212) 245-4639, fax.: (212) 765-4197

Δ Moss, Dr. Ralph W.: **The Cancer Industry - the classic exposé on the cancer establishment** (U.S.A., 1980) (ISBN 1-55778-439-6) Paragon House, 90 Fifth Avenue, New York, NY 10011, U.S.A., tél.: (212) 620-2820

Δ Santé et Bien-Etre Canada: **Compte rendu du Colloque de la F.O.R.C.T.C. sur l'épidémiologie du cancer** (Canada, 1992) (ISSN 0228-8702)

magazines

Δ **Scientific American** (January 1994)

Δ **Time** (April 1994)

Immunity

Δ Douglas-Hume, Ethyl: **Pasteur or Béchamp ? - a lost chapter in the history of biology** (England, 1947) C.W. Daniel Company, Saffron Walden, Essex, England

Δ Nonclerg, Marie: **Antoine Béchamp - l'homme et le savant** (France, 1982) (ISBN 2-224-00854-6) Maloine Éditeur, 27 rue de l'École-de-Médecine, 75006, Paris, France

magazine

Δ Saturday Night - article: **Blood Feud** (Canada, December 1992)

REALIZATION

Δ   Bach, Richard: **The Reluctant Messiah** (U.S.A., 1977) (ISBN 2-08-064014-3)

Δ   Carter, Dr. James P.: **Racketeering in Medicine - the suppression
    of alternatives** (U.S.A., 1992) (ISBN 1-878901-32-X)
    Hamptons Roads Publishing, 891 Norfolk Square, Norfolk VA 23502
    Tél.: (804) 459-2453, fax.: (804) 455-8907

Δ   Center for Self-Governance: **It's Your Health So Take Charge - informed
    choices for a healthy nation** (U.S.A., 1993) (ISBN 1-55815-282-2)
    Institute for Contemporary Studies, San Francisco, CA 94102, U.S.A.
    Tél.: (800) 326-0263

Δ   Foundation For Inner Peace: **A Course in Miracles** (text, manual for teachers
    and workbook for students) (U.S.A., 1975) (ISBN 0-9606388-0-6)
    Foundation for Inner Peace, P.O.Box 635, Tiburon, CA 94920, U.S.A.

Δ   Greenberg, Dr. Michael A.: **Off the Pedestal - transforming the business
    of medicine** (U.S.A., 1990) (ISBN 0-942540-39-5)
    Breakthru Publishing, P.O. Box 2866, Houston, TX 77252-2866, U.S.A.
    Tél.: (713) 522-7660

Δ   Mongeau, Serge: **Parce que la paix n'est pas une utopie**
    (Québec, 1990) (ISBN 2-89111-406-X)
    Collection Paix/Libre Expression, 2016 rue St-Hubert, Montréal H2L 3Z5

Δ   Nozick, Marcia: **No Place Like Home - Building sustainable communities**
    (Canada, 1992) (ISBN 0-88810-415-4) Canadian Council on Social Development,
    55 Parkdale Avenue, Ottawa, K1Y 4G1, tel.: (613) 728-1865

Δ   Robard, Isabelle: **La santé assassinée** (France, 1992) (ISBN 2-908986-11-6)
    Éditions de l'Ancre, 9-11 rue Benoît-Malon, 92156 Suresnes Cedex, France

Δ   Small Wright, Machaelle: **Behaving As If God In All Life Mattered**
    (U.S.A., 1983) (ISBN 0-9617713-0-5)
    Perelandra Ltd, P.O.Box 3603, Warrenton, VA 22186, U.S.A.

magazine

Δ   UTNE Reader articles: **Managed Care Scam** (U.S.A., Sept.-Oct. 1994)

INVITATION

You've enjoyed this book...

Why not share your experience and take advantage of interesting rebates when reserving a number of copies for your friends and neighbors on the same order.

Turn the page for savings of up to 40% off the cover price for ten and more copies.

You may want to use one of the order forms on the following pages and return it to us by mail.

Thank you and lots of success in your new endeavor!

PRICE LIST

IN THE USA

Prices per book for the following number of copies ON THE SAME ORDER:

Number of books	1 - 4	5 - 9	10 or more
Cover price	$14.95	$14.95	$14.95
Rebate	0%	20%	40%
Price per book	$14.95	$11.95	$8.95
+ S&H			
Total price per book	**$17.00**	**$14.00**	**$11.00**

Please make your cheque or money order payable to HERE'S THE KEY INC.

Our sales office address is:

Here's The Key Inc.
P.O. Box 223
Morgan, VT 05853

To reach us by fax or telephone simply dial:

Fax: 1- 802-895-4669 • Tel: 1- 802-895-4914

IN CANADA

Prices per book for the following number of copies ON THE SAME ORDER:

Number of books	1 - 4	5 - 9	10 or more
Cover price	$19.95	$19.95	$19.95
Rebate	0%	20%	40%
Price per book	$19.95	$15.95	$11.95
+ GST and S&H			
Total price per book	**$23.00**	**$19.00**	**$15.00**

Please make your cheque or money order payable to HERE'S THE KEY INC.

Our sales office address is:

Here's The Key Inc.
P.O. Box 113
Coaticook, QC
J1A 2S9

To reach us by fax or telephone simply dial:

Fax: 1-819-835-5433 • Tel: 1-819-835-9520

GIFT ORDER FORM: *The Medical Mafia*

Send one copy as a gift in my name

to

Name: _____

Address: _____ Apt.: _____

City: _____ State-Prov: _____ ZIP-Postal code: _____

from

Name: _____

Address: _____ Apt.: _____

City: _____ State-Prov: _____ ZIP-Postal code: _____

Enclosed is my ☐ cheque ☐ money order

for: ☐ In the USA = $17.00
☐ In Canada = $23.00

GIFT ORDER FORM: *The Medical Mafia*

Send one copy as a gift in my name

to

Name: _____

Address: _____ Apt.: _____

City: _____ State-Prov: _____ ZIP-Postal code: _____

from

Name: _____

Address: _____ Apt.: _____

City: _____ State-Prov: _____ ZIP-Postal code: _____

Enclosed is my ☐ cheque ☐ money order

for: ☐ In the USA = $17.00
☐ In Canada = $23.00

Here's The Key Inc.
P.O. Box 223, Morgan, VT 05853
P.O. Box 113, Coaticook, QC J1A 2S9

Here's The Key Inc.
P.O. Box 223, Morgan, VT 05853
P.O. Box 113, Coaticook, QC J1A 2S9

ORDER FORM: *The Medical Mafia*

_____ copies @ $_____.00 per book = $_____.00

Enclosed is my ☐ cheque ☐ money order

Name: _____

Address: _____ Apt.: _____

City: _____ State-Prov: _____ ZIP-Postal code: _____

ORDER FORM: *The Medical Mafia*

_____ copies @ $_____.00 per book = $_____.00

Enclosed is my ☐ cheque ☐ money order

Name: _____

Address: _____ Apt.: _____

City: _____ State-Prov: _____ ZIP-Postal code: _____

ORDER FORM: *The Medical Mafia*

_____ copies @ $_____.00 per book = $_____.00

Enclosed is my ☐ cheque ☐ money order

Name: _____

Address: _____ Apt.: _____

City: _____ State-Prov: _____ ZIP-Postal code: _____

ORDER FORM: *The Medical Mafia*

_____ copies @ $_____.00 per book = $_____.00

Enclosed is my ☐ cheque ☐ money order

Name: _____

Address: _____ Apt.: _____

City: _____ State-Prov: _____ ZIP-Postal code: _____

Here's The Key Inc.
P.O. Box 223, Morgan, VT 05853
P.O. Box 113, Coaticook, QC J1A 2S9

Here's The Key Inc.
P.O. Box 223, Morgan, VT 05853
P.O. Box 113, Coaticook, QC J1A 2S9

Here's The Key Inc.
P.O. Box 223, Morgan, VT 05853
P.O. Box 113, Coaticook, QC J1A 2S9

Here's The Key Inc.
P.O. Box 223, Morgan, VT 05853
P.O. Box 113, Coaticook, QC J1A 2S9

NOTES